IN SEARCH OF
HEALTH

Exploring Alternatives in Medicine

IN SEARCH OF
HEALTH

MICHAEL VOLEN, M.D.

Gateway Press
Mill Valley, California

Gateway Press
P.O. Box 5180
Mill Valley, California 94942

First Printing: April 1986.
Editor: Kimberley Peterson
Cover design: Kathleen Vande Kieft
Design and coordination: Matrix Productions
Typesetting: Mackenzie-Harris Corp., San Francisco, CA
Cover Photo: Spiral Galaxy M-83
Copyright Dr. Reginald J. Dufour, Rice University

Printed in the United States of America

LIBRARY OF CONGRESS CATALOGING-IN-PUBLICATION DATA

Volen, Michael P., 1944–
   In search of health.

   Bibliography: p.
   1. Self-care, Health.   2. Therapeutic systems.
I. Title.   [DNLM: 1. Alternative Medicine—popular works.   2. Self Care—popular works.   WB 120 V914i]
RA776.95.V64   1986   613   85-30239
ISBN 0-936533-00-5 (pbk.)

To my parents
Irving and Edith Volen

Acknowledgments

No book is the work of a single individual, and I wish to acknowledge the many teachers, past and present, who have contributed to my own understanding of health and medicine. I also wish to express my appreciation of the friends who have supported me in the preparation of this book. Special thanks are due Merrill and Kimberley Peterson for editorial help, as well as general coordination of book design and production.

Contents

Preface   5
Prologue   7

PART ONE: DOCTORS AND PATIENTS TODAY

1   Modern Medicine: Strengths and Weaknesses   14
2   The Diseases of Civilization   29
3   The Meaning of Illness   43
4   Symptoms as Symbol   58
5   Muscles, Emotions, and Illness   72
6   Avoiding the Hazards of Modern Medicine   86

PART TWO: EXPLORING ALTERNATIVES IN MEDICINE

7   Hypnosis, Suggestion, and the Process of Healing   106
8   Perspectives on Healing: East and West   121
9   Acupuncture and Western Medicine   135
10 Man's Natural Diet   151
11 Protecting Your Personal Health   169
12 Medicine for the Future   183

Annotated Bibliography   199

Preface

During fifteen years as a practicing physician, I have had the opportunity to help care for patients in various settings, ranging from hospital Emergency Rooms to University clinics to private practice. Throughout this time, I have been consistently impressed by the fact that many medical problems could have been entirely prevented if people had taken greater responsibility for their health. Often, this could have been accomplished by adopting a healthier lifestyle and diet, as well as learning to listen to the message in the symptoms of illness.

When people become sick, it is often an indication that certain physical or emotional changes are needed. Typically, these changes cannot be accomplished by a doctor, but can only be made by the individual. Yet the medical care that people receive too often concentrates only on treating the obvious symptoms of illness. It ignores the need for changes that will respond to the real causes of the illness.

This realization left me frustrated with the nature of medical care today and provided the impetus for this book. *In Search of Health* examines how any individual can take greater responsibility for his or her health and help to avoid serious illness. In addition, *In Search of*

Health evaluates our current medical system—how it works, and how it does *not* work—offering alternative approaches to health care that could more effectively meet people's needs.

Much of the book is drawn from my own experience as a physician. The stories of patients are based on real events, but the names and specific circumstances have been changed to protect the identities of those involved.

A good deal in this book is critical of what doctors do; however, this criticism is not meant as an attack upon the medical profession. I feel privileged to be a part of this profession, and my intention is to suggest how doctors could be more successful in accomplishing their true purpose—helping their patients to get well.

I believe we have the knowledge and the capability to be far healthier, both as individuals and as a society, than we are today. However, for this to happen we need to confront those habits and patterns in our lives that cause our illnesses. We must also broaden our perspective on health care to allow certain approaches to treatment, now considered unconventional, to become more a part of our medical system.

It is my hope that this book will help readers achieve a higher level of personal health and well-being. Perhaps it may also serve as a stimulus for physicians and other health professionals to make their own interaction with patients more satisfying.

Prologue

It was a late October day in New England. The last summer visitors from the city were gone, and for the first time the air hinted at the piercing cold of the coming winter. Even the quality of the light was changed: the bright, thin sunlight no longer warmed as it had throughout the summer months. Most of the leaves had fallen from the trees, and now rustled in the streets in brown drifts when the wind blew, while branches stood bare against a blue sky. A sense of quiet hung over the town, as though it were somehow turned in upon itself as all its inhabitants prepared for the onset of winter.

The quiet even extended to the hospital Emergency Room where I was on duty. It had been an uneventful day with only a trickle of patients to be seen, and by eleven o'clock that night the Emergency Room was silent and empty. It was time to retire for some sleep while I had the opportunity. Every four days I worked a twenty-four hour shift, which could become exhausting toward the end if we had remained busy during the night. But on a night like this, I thought hopefully, I might even be fortunate enough to sleep undisturbed until morning.

However, this was not to be. At three o'clock I was roused from a deep sleep by the familiar ring of the telephone beside the bed, and the night shift nurse informed me there was a patient to be seen. This was one of the hardest parts of work in the Emergency Room: no matter how exhausted I might be, I must become immediately awake and alert, and be prepared to deal properly with whatever sort of problem presented itself.

Often the problems that appeared in the middle of the night were not the most pleasant. It was not unusual to enter the Emergency Room and discover a drunken, perhaps combative, accident victim, covered with blood from gashes in his head that must somehow be stitched together properly despite his lack of cooperation.

Fortunately the patient tonight did not sound too bad. The nurse had told me it was a man who had been struck by a car while riding a bicycle, but he did not appear seriously hurt. I rubbed the sleep from my eyes and muttered to myself about the kind of fool who would be out riding a bicycle in the middle of a cold October night. I walked down the hall to the Emergency Room, feeling grouchy and irritable at being awakened to care for a problem caused by someone's irresponsible behavior.

When I arrived, I found something very different from what I had expected. Seated on an examination table in one of the treatment rooms was a cheerful, robust-looking man. His chart said he was seventy-five years old, but he looked much younger. He greeted me pleasantly, and assured me that he had nothing more than a few bruises, but that the police had insisted on his coming to be examined. As I checked him over and confirmed that he was not hurt, he told me his story.

He was the sexton of a church in a small town at the other end of the state. He lived alone in a room in the church and worked as a caretaker. His bicycle was his only means of transportation. Every year at this time, for many years, he traveled to visit an old friend who lived in this part of the state. This journey took him the better part of twenty-four hours on his bicycle. He was in the habit of simply pedaling through the night, as he had been doing tonight, to reach his destination. This was the first time, he told me, that anything had happened to interrupt his trip, and he was more concerned with the damage to his bicycle than with any injury to himself.

It appeared that his bicycle would need some repairs before he could proceed any further, and while he was sorry to be delayed, he took the whole situation with good humor. He was not upset that he had been hit by a car or that his bicycle was damaged, but simply accepted what had happened. Indeed, he projected a sense of internal peacefulness that seemed to allow him to face whatever might occur with the same easy acceptance. I was impressed by the spirit of this man, as well as his physical appearance.

His face had a ready smile and his body was lean and spare; he could easily have passed for a man twenty years younger. His legs in particular were hard as tree limbs, and were covered with thick, ropy muscles from long miles of bicycling. Although he was nearly fifty years my senior, I doubted that I could keep up with him for long in any kind of physical activity. He was altogether very different from what we expect a person of seventy-five years to be, and I felt fortunate to have made his acquaintance. He seemed a truly *healthy* person in the fullest sense of the word.

Such people are not often encountered today, especially in the Emergency Room of a hospital. The Emergency Room provides abundant opportunities to see the less pleasant sides of human behavior, so it was a refreshing change to find a man who represented such a state of positive health.

I agreed I could find nothing more than some minor bruises, and wished him good luck with the remainder of his trip. As I returned to bed, I realized that my bad humor at being awakened had vanished entirely. Instead, I felt uplifted by my encounter with this unusual man. Although he had been brought to the hospital to receive help, I felt he had done far more for me in our brief meeting than I had done for him.

With no explicit intention on his part, he was able to act as a teacher for anyone prepared to learn from him. And his teaching was on the most profound level—that of personal example. Through his own behavior, he demonstrated the capacity of a person to maintain a very high level of physical and emotional health, even at what today is considered to be "old age." Although it was more than ten years ago that I met him, I like to think that he is still pedaling his bicycle down the back roads of New England.

Most people of any age, let alone those in their seventies, could not imagine hopping on their bicycle and pedaling two hundred miles to visit a friend. Many of us, especially older people, simply do not believe that we are capable of such activity. We assume that growing older is inevitably associated with deterioration of the body; we are no longer good for much over age sixty-five. This destructive belief can become a self-fulfilling prophecy, because once we give up doing things it is not long before we do, in fact, lose the ability to do them.

The man in the Emergency Room obviously did not have such beliefs about what he could no longer do. He had simply continued to ride his bicycle, regardless of his age. It was no accident that he could pedal all day; it came from taking proper care of his body. People like this not only provide inspiration, but also serve as a practical model for just how this can be done.

In examining individuals who live to a healthy and robust old age, certain patterns become apparent. I once read an article describing a study of people in China who had lived to be a hundred or more. The purpose of the study was to discover whether these people shared any common behaviors that might explain their longevity. Much detailed scientific data exists on the subject of longevity, but this article got right to the heart of the matter.

This study concluded that three principles, if followed, provided the best chance to live to a healthy old age: first—eat a diet of simple, natural, unprocessed foods; second—get plenty of exercise, especially walking, on a regular basis; and third—avoid getting angry. That was it.

The people in this study, who lived mainly in small villages in the mountains of China, may have found it easier to abide by these principles than most people in modern America. But the article still touched upon a basic truth that applies to people anywhere. While undoubtedly an oversimplification of a complex subject, its conclusions made a lot of sense. They had identified the same three primary factors in determining health that I encounter repeatedly in my own medical practice.

These are diet, emotional state, and physical condition of the individual. People typically get sick because they do not eat properly, because they do not take proper physical care of their bodies, and especially because they are experiencing emotional stress in their lives. Often elements of all three are involved, and each can reinforce the others. Poor nutrition will make you more susceptible to stress, while the worse you feel emotionally, the less likely you are to pay enough attention to eating properly or exercising. This in turn leads to further stress. The result is a self-reinforcing negative spiral that may eventually lead to illness.

However, it is possible for anyone to exert some control in all of these areas. We all have the capacity to decide what food we eat, how we care for our bodies—whether we exercise, get enough sleep, smoke cigarettes, drink too much alcohol, and so on—and, at least to some extent, what emotional states we experience. Each person can choose between a lifestyle likely to lead to illness or one more consistent with a longer and healthier life. Although it is never possible to control all the variables, we can at least do our best to create the level of health we want. While we may not all be bicycling through the night at age seventy-five, we can certainly make the most of our body's potential.

PART ONE

DOCTORS AND PATIENTS
TODAY

1

Modern Medicine
Strengths and Weaknesses

Technological Medicine

The Emergency Room is the nerve center of a hospital. As a medical student, I was always attracted to its air of unpredictable excitement. Thus, it was no surprise that my first job as a doctor was in a hospital Emergency Room. The hospital was in a small New England town that slumbered peacefully through most of the year, and then, for a few short months in the summer, became a bustling seaside resort. The Emergency Room reflected the changing seasons—often quiet in winter, while swamped in summer with vacationers suffering from cuts, sunburns, and fishhooks stuck in their fingers. It was never the same from one day to the next, which invariably made it an interesting place to work.

Hours of near boredom, when nothing seemed to happen, could suddenly turn into the frantic activity of dealing with multiple emergencies at the same time. One never knew quite what the distant wail of the ambulance sirens would bring, or what sort of problem would come through the doors at the next moment.

This element of surprise contributed to the fascination of the Emergency Room, but it also made it challenging to work there. Although I became accustomed to a variety of odd situations, I never entirely lost the feeling that one day I might be confronted with a problem too catastrophic to manage properly.

However, there was much about this work that was very satisfying. Often, as I sat alone in the hospital at night, I experienced the curious sensation of knowing that, should anything happen to one of the forty thousand or so people in the surrounding towns, I would be the person first called upon to help. And often I *was* able to help. I saw people in difficult, sometimes highly unusual, circumstances, and many times the treatment I was able to provide had a real impact on their lives.

On a few occasions, I even saved some lives. I recall resuscitating a man who had suffered a cardiac arrest—pushing rhythmically on his chest to keep the blood flowing, attaching electrical leads to shock his heart back into life, snapping out orders for drugs to be injected, the intense concentration and controlled urgency in each moment—and later seeing him regain consciousness and awaken to go on with his life. I also recall an astute diagnosis of meningitis in a little girl who seemed just a bit too sick for the flu—first making the difficult decision to perform a spinal tap in the Emergency Room, and when the diagnosis was confirmed, rushing her to the nearest medical center for more sophisticated treatment than we could provide in our small hospital.

These were very gratifying experiences for me. They also fit a certain pattern. After spending some time in the Emergency Room, I realized that the people who were really helped there had certain things in common. For the most part, they were people whose problems could be addressed on a largely mechanical level, and usually they needed something done for them immediately.

One of my most compelling memories of such a situation is of the first patient I treated for a dislocated shoulder. While working on his house he had fallen off a ladder, landing on his shoulder. The force of his fall had wrenched the humerus, the long bone of the upper arm, from its socket at the shoulder joint. When he arrived at the Emergency Room, his shoulder had a most alarming appearance: it was strikingly deformed and the slightest attempt at movement caused him a great deal of pain. The patient was a big, muscular man, but his face was pale, and his expression as he looked down at his arm was one of mingled terror and disbelief.

He was extremely reluctant to let me touch his shoulder, but the only way it could be fixed was by popping the bone back into the socket through steady pressure on the extended arm. Although I *had* never done this myself, I had watched other doctors. Something clearly needed to be done immediately, and as nobody more experienced was available, I coaxed him onto the table and very carefully took hold of his arm.

Slowly I increased the force until I was pulling with every bit of my strength. I could sense him trying to cooperate but he was unable to overcome the involuntary resistance into which his own muscles were locked. I pulled until I could feel the sweat running down my body. Just as I began to wonder how much longer I could continue, there was at last a moment of relaxation. With an audible pop the shoulder slipped back into place. Suddenly the pain was gone and the fear in his face was replaced by a wonderful expression of enormous relief. We wrapped his arm in a sling, gave him some instructions for further care, and sent him home full of gratitude.

This was what medicine was supposed to be like. The patient had a problem, the doctor fixed it, and that was the end of the matter. When problems in the Emergency Room could be dealt with in this way as purely mechanical disorders, then people could really be helped. And those who were helped the most were those with the most serious mechanical malfunction.

The man who suffers a heart attack, the accident

victim with multiple injuries, the patient with a drug overdose—in such situations the life-support systems of the body are acutely and severely compromised. The body is unable to cope with what is happening unassisted. If the person is to survive, some form of external intervention is necessary.

Modern medicine works at its best under such circumstances; this is where the powerful drugs and technology available in the hospital find their most appropriate use. The doctor is dealing only with fundamental life functions—breath, heartbeat, circulation—so it is possible to strip away all the complexities of mind and emotion that otherwise play so great a role in the condition of the patient. For problems that can be approached this way, the technology of modern medicine is highly effective; there is no better place to appreciate this than in the Emergency Room.

Limitations of Medical Technology

While I felt a real satisfaction at being able to apply this technology myself, I gradually became aware of other aspects of the Emergency Room that were less satisfying. One of these was the realization that people did not just appear in the Emergency Room for no reason. Invariably there were causes for whatever was wrong with them, and often these causes turned out to be complex and of some duration.

A man in the Emergency Room with a heart attack, for example, was not there simply because of something that had happened that day. The actual heart attack was only the final step in a process that had begun long ago and had inevitably led to this moment in the Emergency Room. Deposits of fat had been forming in his arteries for many years, slowly increasing in size and narrowing the blood vessels. Eventually, one of the arteries to the heart had become so blocked that all blood flow ceased, and he experienced the catastrophic event we call a heart attack.

The man with a heart attack might be followed by a woman in diabetic coma, another common Emergency Room situation. Again, it was my job to see the patient through the crisis, administering appropriate drugs and intravenous fluids to correct her biochemical imbalance. The response to this treatment was usually successful and very gratifying. But while it was important to provide this care, I also realized that this crisis, too, was a complication of a chronic disease. Had the real causes of this disease been addressed earlier, then perhaps this woman might not have found herself in the Emergency Room.

Although I was only required to help these patients through an acute crisis, I could not help but realize that the crisis might have been prevented by dealing with its underlying causes earlier in their lives. As I saw one patient after another who fit this pattern, it became evident how many problems could have been prevented at an earlier stage, had the necessary steps been taken. These steps often involved quite straightforward changes in lifestyle and diet, but for some reason they were ignored in the medical care that people received.

If large numbers of people are going to experience heart attacks or other life-threatening illnesses, then we need well-equipped Emergency Rooms to take care of them. But clearly it would be far better to prevent these illnesses in the first place. Yet our medical system seems to be structured so that, as doctors, we do little until a disease reaches some point of crisis. Only then do we step in with our powerful technology to try to rescue the patient as best we can.

Eventually, I came to feel that while work in the Emergency Room could be highly rewarding, much of the time we *were* trying to put the pieces back together after the damage had already been done. Even when we were successful at seeing someone through a crisis, this did not mean the problem was at an end. The man who is fortunate enough to get to a hospital in time to survive his heart attack is still not cured of heart disease. Unless significant changes are made, the same conditions that led to his heart attack will continue to create further symptoms of illness and perhaps even another heart attack. Thus, there were clear limits to what we could accomplish for such a patient through technological intervention alone.

These limitations were not the only frustrations associated with the Emergency Room. When a patient with a heart attack arrives at the hospital complaining of chest pain, one may speculate about how this crisis might have been averted, but it is at least clear what must be done for him now. However, most people who come to the Emergency Room with chest pain are *not* having a heart attack. They may be worried that this is happening, but far more often they are experiencing muscle spasms, indigestion, or, most often, anxiety.

When such people came to the Emergency Room, I wondered what could be done for them. They were not experiencing a medical emergency that required intervention, but their problem was still real. They had come to the Emergency Room because something was wrong and they needed help. My assurances that they were not having a heart attack were invariably welcome, but my medical training seemed to have little else to offer; I had only been taught to prescribe some kind of drug. If they had muscle spasm, I was to prescribe a muscle relaxant, while if it was a digestive problem, I might give them an antispasmodic medication. And if the problem was anxiety or emotional stress, I could give them a tranquilizer.

I found these treatments unsatisfactory. Handing out various pills to everyone who came through the Emergency Room might suppress the most obvious symptoms, but this approach did not address whatever was causing these symptoms. Many patients had already received such treatment from other doctors. Often, they were taking medications that had been ineffective or that had even created new problems through undesirable side effects. I was shocked when I first realized what a large proportion of people were regularly taking medications, and how many different kinds were taken by some of them.

I found myself spending more time trying to get people off unnecessary drugs than prescribing new ones. Drugs might be highly effective in certain emergency situations, but they would not solve most of the routine health problems I saw. However, while I knew another prescription was not the answer, I did not know what else to offer instead.

Health: Mapping the Territory

My experiences in the Emergency Room made me wish to understand what sort of health care would really help people to resolve their illness. To do this, it was necessary to look at some questions about the nature of health and illness.

Why do people get sick? What is the significance of their symptoms? And what is the appropriate response to these symptoms so that the patient can regain a state of health? These questions should be fundamental to any practice of medicine. They are difficult and complex, but the fascination of medicine lies in gaining a more complete understanding of their answers.

This process may lead in unexpected directions. In my case, it has taken me a long way from what is accepted today as conventional medical practice. This has not been out of an intention to seek out the unconventional, but has simply been the consequence of trying to understand what patients really need. The solutions to this problem are often not provided in regular medical training and one is obliged to look elsewhere.

Although medicine today is extremely sophisticated, it

operates from a perspective that can be quite limited. Human beings tend to be seen as complicated biochemical mechanisms, and are treated as such when anything goes wrong. Usually this treatment consists of drugs or surgery. The doctor may prescribe a drug to correct his patient's symptoms, or if this does not work, he may eventually resort to cutting out whatever part of the body is not functioning properly. This approach may work well in the Emergency Room, but when it is applied to ongoing health care the result is less satisfactory.

Our medical system can be thought of as a map that charts the territory of health and illness. Like any map, its purpose is to help you find your way around the territory it describes. However, no map, no matter how well constructed, can ever be the same as the reality it represents.

If you are driving in a car, a road map will guide you to your destination. However, if you are flying in an airplane, a map that shows only the roads will be much less useful, and if you are walking where there are no roads, it will be almost worthless. You will need a different sort of map to find your way.

In the same way that some maps show roads, while others show rivers and mountains, there can also be different maps of the human organism. The map provided by modern medicine emphasizes only certain aspects of the reality that it represents. It provides a highly detailed description of human anatomy and physiology, and when used for this purpose it can be an excellent guide. However, the error we often make is to assume that this particular map is a complete representation of reality, for in doing so we ignore the features that have been left out. We also forget that there can be other maps of the same territory. These maps are not incorrect, but simply emphasize different features, and at times it is appropriate to consult them for a more complete picture.

It is exciting to realize that such different maps exist, and that they may reveal connections between the presence of an illness and events in the patient's life that may not be recognized by conventional medicine. Thus, our medical system is not wrong; it has simply become locked into a perspective that recognizes only part of a much larger picture. This has resulted in certain assumptions about health and illness that are not necessarily valid, and do not contribute to providing the most effective treatment. One of these assumptions is that illness is something external to the patient, rather than intimately related to circumstances in that person's life. This thinking has become so firmly embedded that it is easy to forget it is only an assumption. It is even reflected in our language.

An illness is a thing you "have" or "get," as though it is something external that you have acquired. We speak of "getting" a cold or "catching" a cold, suggesting that colds are somehow floating around invisibly in the environment. The implicit assumption is that when we become sick, it is because we have had the misfortune to come into contact with one of these airborne colds. Thus, patterns of speech reflect the common perception of both doctor and patient that illness is a consequence of some external influence.

In the case of a cold or other infectious disease, it is true that there really is something in the environment: these are submicroscopic particles, far smaller than a single cell, that we refer to as viruses. These viruses appear to be associated with certain illnesses, including the common cold. The virus is commonly considered the "cause" of the cold, but the actual cause-and-effect relationship between the two is considerably more complex.

Although viruses are all around us, we do not develop a cold every time we come in contact with them. If a group of people is exposed to cold viruses, a few will come down with bad colds, some will experience a mild illness, and some will not get sick at all. Obviously, more than mere exposure to a virus is involved in "catching" a cold.

The complex process by which every individual interacts with his or her surroundings must also be considered. We refer to this process as our individual "resistance" or "immune response." When in good health, we may, for the most part, be unaware of its continual activity. However, when this process fails and we become sick, we are reminded of how much we depend upon it to protect us.

How each person reacts to a cold virus, or to any other microorganism, will be influenced by what is happening in his or her life. People experience illness, including colds, when they are stressed, when they have been eating poorly, when they are unhappy, and especially when a number of these conditions exist at the same time. Under these conditions, an internal state is created in which illness can more easily develop, and the stage is set for some external factor, such as a particular virus, to stimulate the condition we refer to as "having a cold." However, if we blame the illness entirely on the virus, we will miss the point of why it occurred and what we really need to do about it.

A cold often indicates that you are overtired, poorly nourished, or unduly stressed. The symptoms, although uncomfortable, are a way of remedying these conditions by making you pay attention to your own needs. However, people usually feel they do not have time to be sick, but must continue their usual routine despite the illness.

Thus, the typical response to a cold is to treat it with a pill. We have an enormous industry devoted to marketing pills that suppress the most troublesome symptoms and allow us to go about our business. To the extent that they are successful, they actually allow us to ignore all those things in our life that made us get sick in the first place.

Drug companies are now at work on a new kind of drug that would not just suppress the symptoms of a cold, but actually destroy the cold virus and provide a real "cure." If such a drug is ever developed, it is sure to be an enormous commercial success. It will undoubtedly be hailed as another "miracle of modern medicine" and enthusiastically embraced by millions of people. And I must admit that the existence of a pill that could make a cold disappear without a trace would be difficult to resist.

But I wonder about the ultimate effect of having such a drug available. Perhaps it would prove to be more of a disaster than a benefit. What would happen if, every time you felt the first signs of a cold, you could swallow a pill and make them disappear immediately? We can only speculate, of course, but it is possible that by continually suppressing the actual appearance of a cold, any underlying problems, such as a need for rest or a better diet, would never be addressed. Instead of getting at least some attention during the course of a minor illness, these problems would remain unresolved, and continue to grow until they found some other form of expression that would prove a good deal more devastating than a simple cold.

Defining Illness: Structure Versus Function

Infectious diseases, with their model of illness as caused by a specific external agent, tend to serve as a prototype for thinking about disease of all kinds. However, when we attempt to relate this model to other forms of illness, it becomes even less applicable. We say that someone "gets" an ulcer, or arthritis, or cancer, although just what it is that he "gets" is even less clear than in the case of the cold. Yet again, there is the assumption that the illness comes from outside the person and its cause is somehow separate from him.

This perspective also influences how we think about what happens when a person is sick. What does it mean, for example, to say that someone "has" an ulcer? We tend to define the problem as the actual physical presence of an ulcer in the lining of the intestine; in other words, the ulcer *is* the disease, and treatment is directed at removing it. Make the ulcer go away, whether by suppressing it with a drug or cutting it out surgically, and the problem is eliminated.

This is not necessarily wrong, and this approach will help some people, but it is not the only way to define the problem. By defining the disease as the ulcer itself, we see it as essentially a *structural* problem—something is wrong with the patient's physical structure that must be corrected. However, it is also possible to view the illness as a *functional* problem. From this perspective, the ulcer is no longer something external that the patient "got;" it is the result of some dysfunction in the body. Therefore, it can be treated not only by trying to remove it directly, but also by correcting the underlying dysfunction.

This is a crucial distinction. The current medical approach concentrates on the obvious structural manifestations of illness—an ulcer, a tumor, an infection—but often ignores the underlying functional disturbance that led to their appearance. When the goal is seen simply as removal of "disease," the doctor may be led to treat the ulcer, rather than the person who has it. However, if illness is perceived as a dysfunction of the entire organism, the doctor is obliged to pay attention to the condition of the whole person.

Ulcers are produced in part by inappropriate secretion of acid by the stomach, and are usually treated with drugs that counteract this process. Some of the drugs recently developed for this purpose have become among the most widely prescribed medications in this country. They have been hailed as major breakthroughs in ulcer treatment, and are prescribed for millions of people today at a cost approaching a billion dollars a year.

While many people have undoubtedly been helped by these medications, it is not unreasonable to ask what these drugs accomplish. They suppress acid production to allow faster healing of the ulcer, which is certainly worthwhile, but they do not change the overall condition of the patient. Although this drug therapy may help the symptoms, it is not the same thing as resolving the illness.

When the drug is stopped, it is not unusual for symptoms to return. This is not surprising because nothing has altered the original causes of the ulcer. And if the symptoms do return, the patient is told by his doctor that he must go back on medication again.

While such treatment is clearly better than doing nothing, and is sometimes necessary, the real concern is correcting the underlying dysfunction. We know that the stomach's production of acid is controlled by the autonomic nervous system. This is the part of the nervous system that regulates functions of the body that are not usually under voluntary control. Like many other medical problems, the excessive acid production involved in ulcer disease can be seen as a sign of autonomic imbalance or dysfunction.

Because the autonomic nervous system is sensitive to physical, emotional, and nutritional influences, a variety of factors such as poor diet or emotional stress can contribute to an imbalance. Thus, anything that restores autonomic balance might be considered a possible treatment. These possibilities are numerous, and in the case of a peptic ulcer, may range from stress reduction techniques, to changes in diet, to treatment with acupuncture.

This approach entails not only diagnosing an ulcer and prescribing medication, but examining the physical and emotional condition of the whole person. It presumes the physician will be concerned with a much wider area of the patient's life. However, this step is not usually taken in our medical system. Whether the problem is a peptic ulcer or some other condition, it is typically defined primarily in structural terms. This is often due to the fact that doctors are good at fixing structural problems. Faced with a broken bone to be set, or a tumor to be removed, the modern physician knows exactly how to proceed and can provide his patient with expert care.

This is why our modern medical system is especially impressive in the Emergency Room or Intensive Care Unit, where problems require immediate intervention. However, it is considerably less effective when it comes to treating people with more chronic conditions. And it seems generally incapable of providing help to the enormous number of patients whose physical complaints have a significant emotional or psychological basis.

Taking a New Approach to Health

As a result of our present approach to medicine, physicians today do not provide effective help with many of the common problems presented by their patients. No matter how much money we spend on health care, how many doctors we train, how many hospitals we build, or how many remarkable new medical devices we develop, people are simply not becoming more healthy. The budget for health care steadily climbs to ever more astronomical limits, yet we still experience as much or even more serious disease in our society. This trend will continue until we recognize that what we need is not more of what we already have, but a change in our present approach.

I find more and more people who are reluctant to see a doctor unless it becomes really necessary, because they doubt the doctor will actually do anything that will reach to the root of their problem. For example, one day I received a phone call from a woman who wanted to see me about back pain she had been having. She was a pleasant, well-spoken woman who happened to be a nurse at one of the local hospitals.

She said she had called me because she knew just what her regular doctor would do for her and it was not what she wanted. She said, "He will send me for X-rays and prescribe some pills and I know that is not what I need. I want to know what else can be done to really help me get over this back problem." I have heard essentially the same words from patients a hundred times before. People want treatment that is really going to help them. They are frustrated with standard medical care because often it does not provide this kind of help.

In order to be more effective, it may be necessary to broaden our perspective on what medicine can be. My own practice today includes various techniques not taught in medical school. Some involve no more than common sense and compassion, while others might be considered more esoteric. But more important than the choice of a particular technique is the recognition that medical treatment cannot be directed solely to the removal of symptoms. It must be based on an understanding of why symptoms exist and it must be prepared to address their causes. Working from this premise, a physician can provide his patient with valuable help in resolving an illness.

Illness does not exist in a vacuum. It happens to individual human beings and it can only be fully understood by dealing with it in this context. The failure of modern technological medicine to address this dimension of illness represents its major weakness. In order to correct this, we must change our perspective on how doctors can best provide health care to their patients.

2

The Diseases
of Civilization

The Modern Epidemics

Today, most doctors spend the majority of their time dealing with medical problems that are caused by lifestyle and
diet, and that could have been prevented. This is a relatively new phenomenon. If you had visited a typical hospital in America a hundred years ago, it would have been
quite different from a modern hospital. Not only would it
bear little physical resemblance to today's medical center,
but the hospital's patients would be there for different
reasons. Most of them would have injuries or infectious
diseases; the wards would be filled with people suffering
from tuberculosis, syphilis, pneumonia, infected wounds,
or similar conditions.

If you visit a hospital today, you will still find some
patients with injuries or infections. But most patients will
be hospitalized for complications of heart disease, cancer,
diabetes, hypertension, peptic ulcers, or various other
chronic diseases. These diseases all share something in
common: they are far more widespread than ever before,
and they seem to be associated with Western lifestyles.
This association is so strong that we even refer to them
collectively as "diseases of civilization." They are also

known as "degenerative diseases" because they are not related to any external agent, but are, instead, a degeneration of the body's normal functioning.

The connection between degenerative disease and the lifestyles of Western civilization is increasingly well documented by epidemiological research that examines the patterns of disease among different groups of people. This research reveals that people throughout the world do not have the same medical problems so common to us. In America and other Western societies the major problems are diseases that our recent ancestors did not have, and that people in much of the rest of the world still do not have.

This finding has important implications. If we want to understand why we have a certain disease, there is no better way than to examine people who do *not* have it and determine what they do differently. The entire world provides us with an enormous natural experiment, on a far greater scale than any scientist could devise, to observe the effects of differing lifestyles upon human health. From these observations we know that some people never experience some of our most serious medical problems, even though they are no different from us in a biological sense. What is different is their lifestyle.

Studies of tribal people in South Africa have illustrated how important this difference can be. The people studied still follow their traditional way of life; their diet remains largely unchanged from that of their ancestors. This consists chiefly of roots, grains, and other vegetables. It is very high in starches and other complex carbohydrates, as well as fiber, while very low in fat. It contains no sugar or other processed foods.

While these people have their share of medical problems in the form of infectious diseases and parasites, the chronic degenerative diseases so widespread in the West are notably absent among them. However, it is most interesting that when they move to the cities and abandon

their traditional diet, they begin to develop chronic degenerative diseases.

Perhaps the most striking finding in this research
relates to the incidence of intestinal disease. A visit to any
drugstore in America—with its shelves full of antacids,
digestive aids, laxatives, and hemorrhoid suppositories—
graphically demonstrates how widespread intestinal
complaints are in this country. Yet among tribal peoples,
few experience these problems. Diseases so common in
the West, such as peptic ulcers, hemorrhoids, constipation, diverticulitis, hiatal hernia, and intestinal cancer,
are almost nonexistent among tribal peoples.

In reviewing these studies, I was especially intrigued
to discover appendicitis included on this list. Appendicitis
is not something we usually think of as a degenerative
disease or as being connected to a particular lifestyle. This
illness held a particular interest for me, because I have
experienced it myself. My first visit to a hospital came
when I had my appendix out at age twelve, and I still
remember it quite well.

One pleasant afternoon in early summer, I began to
complain that my stomach hurt. In those days, doctors
still made house calls, and when the pain did not go away,
our family doctor was summoned to examine me. He
pressed my abdomen for a few moments, and then, to my
dismay, pronounced that I had appendicitis and would
have to go to the hospital that night for an operation.

My memories of the time in the hospital are largely
unpleasant: the cold metal surfaces in the operating
room, the black rubber mask on my face, what seemed
like an unreasonably large needle inserted in my arm, and
later, the surprisingly intense pain of the healing incision.
But I survived and the whole experience left no real scars,
other than the one still faintly visible on my abdomen.
What did stay with me was a curiosity about why this had
happened.

When I entered medical school I learned that appendicitis could be a serious condition. If surgery is not performed promptly, the inflamed appendix can rupture, spreading infection throughout the abdominal cavity and leading to major complications and perhaps even death. Though I learned how to diagnose appendicitis, and even participated in several appendectomies, I still did not learn why this happened to people. I did, however, come to appreciate the care I had received. If modern medical care had not been available, my bellyache could well have turned into something a lot more serious, and I might have died of appendicitis when I was twelve years old.

Why do so many people experience this illness? Hundreds of thousands of appendectomies are performed every year. While appendicitis can occur at any age, it primarily afflicts children and young adults who are otherwise in good health. It seems odd that our bodies should be structured in such a way that the appendix, this very inconspicuous and nonessential bit of anatomy, should malfunction so drastically in so many otherwise healthy young people. Some diseases that occur among very young or elderly people tend to single out weaker individuals, but young adulthood is not typically a time for biological selection to take place.

Thus it was something of a relief to realize that appendicitis is not the result of some basic defect in the human organism. Instead, like so many other diseases, it appears to be a consequence of the way we live. While I am grateful to have had a competent surgeon when I was twelve years old, I am glad to know that my appendicitis was most likely the result of being raised on a standard American diet and probably would not have occurred had I eaten differently. Although I would not have thought of it in such terms then, I had my first experience with the diseases of civilization when I was just twelve years old.

Epidemiological studies now suggest that the chief factor contributing to the onset of appendicitis is diet. Yet, despite this evidence, most people, and even most doctors, rarely think of appendicitis as a nutritional problem. Doctors are trained to remove an inflamed appendix, not to inform people how to avoid this condition by eating properly. Yet a change to a more traditional diet, high in fiber and unprocessed foods, and low in fat, could potentially save millions of people from otherwise unnecessary surgery.

The Role of Diet in Preventing Cancer

Appendicitis reflects only one aspect of how diet can affect the digestive system. The diet that can help prevent appendicitis can also protect us from the onslaught of more serious intestinal diseases. Cancer of the colon, or large intestine, is the single most common cancer in America, accounting for fifteen percent of all cases. But among the tribal people in Africa, as well as other less developed cultures around the world, this disease remains quite rare.

Though we are aware of this very important information about intestinal cancer, we do very little with it. We spend millions of dollars on cancer research, while ignoring the straightforward conclusion that the most common form of cancer in this country could be drastically reduced if people would change how they eat. Intestinal cancer occurs even more frequently than lung cancer, yet, while we have extensive programs that warn us of the dangers of smoking, almost nothing is done to warn us about bad eating habits.

Millions of people who would not think of smoking are eating a high-fat, low-fiber diet that will predispose them to intestinal cancer just as surely as smoking cigarettes will predispose them to lung cancer. Unfortunately, this lack of awareness extends to the medical profession. Few doctors today smoke, but most of them consume the same diet as their patients.

One patient with cancer of the colon stands out particularly in my mind. He was a fifty-four-year-old man who had had surgery to remove part of his large intestine after intestinal cancer was diagnosed. The remainder of the intestine ended in a colostomy, an opening in his abdomen to which a plastic bag was attached. He had also received chemotherapy and radiotherapy, and as a side effect of this treatment, his genitals and one leg had permanently swollen to several times their normal size.

Because of this, he required a catheter to collect his urine, and another plastic bag was attached to his leg for this purpose. Despite this treatment, the cancer had continued to spread through his pelvis, and he was in continuing, severe pain for which he required narcotics around the clock. A robust, energetic man who had once run a successful business, he was now too sick to do anything.

He was in very sad condition, and, at this point in the disease, his doctors had nothing left to offer him. Yet all of this need not ever have happened, for his illness could probably have been prevented by a healthier diet. If, twenty years ago, he could have seen a picture of himself as he was now, and known this could be avoided by a change in diet, I believe he would have made whatever change was necessary. But he did *not* know, and he probably assumed his diet was fine. I doubt he ever wondered whether his eating habits might eventually lead him to some terrible disease, and it is unlikely his doctor ever told him.

This sad situation *can* be avoided. We now have information on the direct connection between diet and many serious diseases, and it is essential that people be made aware of it. It is not yet entirely clear how a particular diet might protect against intestinal cancer, but we are beginning to develop some ideas. One theory involves the concept of "intestinal transit time": the time it takes food to pass the length of the intestinal tract. In a typical Western diet, food moves very slowly, while intestinal transit time is much quicker among traditional cultures that consume a high-fiber, low-fat diet.

It appears that a slow transit time may allow harmful waste products to remain in contact with the lining of the intestine for a longer time. Over the years, this continued irritation of the intestine may eventually result in the development of cancer. Because the best stimulus to intestinal transit is bulk, the solution is obvious: an abundance of fiber in the diet is important not only to avoid constipation and allow smooth functioning of the bowels, it is also a possible prevention against intestinal cancer.

Other Diseases of Civilization

The same traditional cultures that are free of intestinal disease are also free of numerous other diseases common in Western societies. A partial list of these includes coronary artery disease, diabetes, hypertension, gall stones, various forms of cancer, as well as peptic ulcers, diverticulitis, and all the other intestinal diseases already mentioned. In addition to cancer of the colon, cancers of the lung, breast, uterus, and prostate, among others, are also more common in the West.

This is clearly an impressive list, but many other diseases could be included here as well. Taken together, they make up the bulk of the medical problems for which people consult doctors today. And to some extent they are almost all preventable.

One factor common to all of these diverse conditions is diet. To function properly, we require a wide variety of nutrients in an appropriate quantity and balance. When these nutrients are not supplied, it is no surprise that our bodies begin to malfunction. However, it is too simple an explanation to attribute all our modern medical problems entirely to diet; other factors are also at work.

One of these is lack of physical exercise. Our bodies are meant to be used regularly, yet it is remarkable just how little exercise we get today. In most of the world, the normal process of daily living demands a good deal of physical exertion. But in Western cultures, the routine of many people has become extremely sedentary. We sit all day at a desk or behind the wheel of a car; thus we must make a point of doing some activity specifically for the exercise it provides. For those who do not do this, illness is often the consequence of bodily weakness and disuse.

Along with improper diet and lack of exercise, another factor affecting our health is environmental pollution. The increasing contamination of our air, food, and water cannot help but affect us in a variety of ways. Many of these effects are subtle and, while not immediately apparent, eventually they take their toll on our health.

All of these factors are relatively new to us: until quite recently, the average person did not have to worry about environmental pollution, adequate exercise, or how to eat a proper diet. The environment had not been significantly affected by industrial technology, exercise was a natural part of life, and food was simple.

Today, these new factors in our lives interact in complex ways to create illnesses that never before existed to the extent they now do. The situation is further compounded by emotional influences that also affect the state of our health. Life in the modern world subjects us to stresses that did not exist in the past, and to which we are not biologically adapted. Constant exposure to noise, crowding, or traffic has a real physical effect upon the body, as does the struggle to find meaningful activity or maintain personal relationships in a complex and rapidly changing world. Our response to this stress is yet another factor to be considered.

Thus the causes of what we call the diseases of civilization are complex. These illnesses are the cumulative manifestation in our bodies of a whole way of living. They have no simple cause to be cured by swallowing a pill, but spring from the very fabric of life in modern society.

In a sense, we have exchanged one set of diseases for another. The social changes that allowed us to control the diseases of a hundred years ago have also created an environment that puts new and different illnesses in their place. Our major medical problems are no longer tuberculosis, malaria, or cholera, as they still are in other parts of the world; instead, we have heart disease, cancer, and diabetes.

These newer problems do not respond to the medical approaches that worked with the old ones. Illnesses caused by lifestyle, diet, and poor habits cannot be resolved through external intervention. Yet this is how our medical system persists in treating them.

Heart Disease: Coronary Bypass or Prevention?

Heart disease is, perhaps, the classic example of degenerative disease and the problems entailed in treating such disease. More specifically referred to as coronary artery disease, it is now the leading cause of death in America. Amazingly, as recently as the last century, coronary artery disease was a relatively uncommon condition accorded just a page or two in medical textbooks. Now, of course, whole books are written on the subject.

Several factors can play a part in this disease, including lack of physical exercise, emotional stress, cigarette smoking, and especially our modern diet of high-fat processed foods. These can all predispose a person to heart disease, although there is some controversy regarding the relative importance of each.

The basic process in this disease is the accumulation of fatty deposits on the walls of the arteries. This takes place throughout the body, but the arteries that supply the heart are particularly vulnerable. As they become narrowed, their capacity to deliver blood to the heart muscle is reduced.

The first sign of coronary artery disease is often experienced as chest pain with exertion, as the narrowed blood vessels are unable to meet the heart's increased demand for blood. Eventually, one of the vessels may become completely blocked so that no blood can flow through it. The portion of heart muscle supplied by this artery actually dies, and this is what we refer to as a heart attack.

Although the precise mechanism is not yet clear, diet seems to be a primary cause of this disease. One factor that has been consistently implicated is the inclusion of large amounts of fat, especially animal fat, in the diet. The problem is compounded by lack of vigorous physical exercise, which leaves the heart muscle with small, poorly developed vessels that are more easily plugged. Cigarette smoking or emotional stress can also contribute to this condition through other biochemical effects.

Because all these factors are amenable to change, coronary artery disease should potentially be a preventable condition. However, our medical system is now focused not so much on preventing these causes, as on treating their results. Various drugs exist to dilate blood vessels, and millions of prescriptions are written for them every year. But while these may be effective in relieving symptoms, they do not change the underlying condition of the heart or the factors that led to this condition.

More drastic treatment may also be considered. In coronary bypass surgery, the narrowed portions of the coronary arteries are replaced by grafts taken from another part of the body. The extraordinary technology involved is a remarkable achievement of our medical system, and every year more of these operations are performed. As this surgery becomes increasingly popular, more sophisticated techniques are being introduced to open plugged coronary arteries.

These surgical techniques are impressive in the skill and coordination of medical resources they require. They are also very expensive. Considering that 150,000 such operations are performed each year, at a conservative estimate of approximately $25,000 per operation, we arrive at a total of around four billion dollars per year spent on coronary bypass surgery. And this number increases every year.

What is actually accomplished at this enormous cost? While bypass surgery directly eliminates the symptoms, it does nothing about the original *cause* of these symptoms. If the patient resumes his old habits of living and eating, he will soon begin to plug up his arteries again, just as he did before. It is estimated that people who have had bypass surgery experience a return of symptoms at the rate of five to fifteen percent per year. The result is that some people may need to return for a second operation, and perhaps even conceivably a third. One recent analysis concluded that soon over half a million people who have had bypass surgery will experience a return of symptoms that may require another operation.

Thus, bypass surgery alone does not seem like the answer to heart disease. No matter how sophisticated the surgery, the problem will not go away until we address what is actually causing it. In the meantime, bypass surgery is a very expensive form of temporary repair; some of the resources devoted to it might be more efficiently used elsewhere.

Recently I saw in the newspaper that a well-known public figure was about to enter the hospital for triple coronary bypass surgery. This means grafts would be made to three separate branches of the arteries to the heart. This surgery is spectacular enough to be reported in the newspaper, and perhaps the surgeons might give this famous man a few more months or years of life.

What is not reported in the newspaper are the people who do *not* go into the hospital for bypass surgery. A person who has made the changes in diet and lifestyle necessary to avoid heart disease is not a dramatic news story. Yet the doctor who helped his patient understand and make these changes has, in a quiet way, accomplished something more impressive and lasting than the most spectacular heart surgery. The small amount of time the doctor devotes to prevention now may save the patient from coronary bypass surgery twenty or thirty years later.

The national statistics regarding heart disease are certainly grim, but it is important to realize that one need not become one of these unfortunate statistics. Coronary artery disease can be prevented, and this prevention ultimately has little to do with doctors or drugs or operations. And this is true not only of heart disease, but of many other serious diseases as well.

Healthy Aging

Many people today find their bodies literally falling apart as they grow older; they are even unable to perform what were once the simplest of tasks. Their muscles become weak and flabby, their joints stiff and painful, their bones thin and brittle. Their heart labors to pump blood and their lungs struggle to move enough air, while digestion becomes erratic and the bowels increasingly sluggish. They find it is an effort to walk a block or to climb a flight of stairs.

Certain changes in the body are inevitable with aging, but growing old does not have to be like this. Much of this deterioration is *not* a natural process, but the consequence of poor diet, inadequate exercise, chronic emotional strain, abuse of cigarettes, alcohol, or drugs, or some other habit that is possible to control and change.

These factors can lead to "degenerative disease" at a surprisingly early age, as in the example of appendicitis in a child, or the heart attacks that Americans in their thirties are now experiencing. But more often the process is slow and gradual; its effects become increasingly apparent as one grows older. While their causes may begin early in life, degenerative diseases usually reach the stage of requiring treatment among older age groups.

Anyone involved in the care of older people cannot

help but be impressed by the ravages of these diseases. I am often saddened when I see signs of chronic disease in the body that are the direct consequence of a lifetime of certain habits. It is particularly sad to realize that these habits are not due to a lack of caring, but are often the result of simply not knowing how to live a natural and healthy life.

As a doctor, I do what I can to help such patients. But while it is never too late to begin to make changes, it is difficult to reverse the cumulative effects of a lifetime. The chronic, degenerative diseases will eventually lead to damage of the body that may be impossible to treat effectively. The only solution is to prevent them from ever reaching this stage.

We have overcome the diseases of the past, but in the process we have developed a new set of illnesses to take their place. However, this exchange is not necessary. It is possible to have the best of both worlds. There is no reason to give up the medical technology that controls diseases that were once serious problems. But we can also retain the elements of a simpler diet and lifestyle to reverse the epidemic of degenerative disease we are now experiencing. This does not mean we must abandon modern civilization and return to living like "primitives." The necessary changes *can* be compatible with modern lifestyles. In fact, increasing numbers of people are already making these changes as they learn to take more responsibility for their health.

If illness in an individual signals the need for some change by that person, then illness that afflicts a whole society suggests that a change in habits must take place on a national level. We are not a healthy society. Our medical problems will not be solved with more doctors or drugs or surgery; they will only be solved by changing how we live.

This conclusion is both frustrating and reassuring. It

is frustrating to realize the limitations of the doctor. Yet, ultimately, it is reassuring that many of the serious medical problems we are likely to encounter today are not inevitable. Some basic, yet relatively simple, changes in our diet and lifestyle could lead to an extraordinary improvement in the physical and emotional health of us all.

3

The Meaning
of Illness

Treating the Patient, Not the Disease

John was a commercial artist in his early thirties who consulted me one day about his blood pressure. He had recently passed a demonstration offering free blood pressure checks and on an impulse had decided to stop. To his surprise, he was told that his blood pressure was higher than it should be and he was advised to see a doctor. He made an appointment with an internist, who agreed that his blood pressure was indeed too high and ordered a chest X-ray, EKG, and various blood and urine tests.

As is usually the case, everything was normal. John was informed by the doctor that he had "essential hypertension," meaning that no specific cause could be found for his elevated blood pressure. He was given a prescription for medication to be taken every day.

The doctor seemed to consider this quite routine, but John was not happy with the outcome. He had always considered himself a healthy person and had never taken medication for any length of time. The idea that he now had to take a pill every day for months or perhaps years, or conceivably even the rest of his life, did not appeal to him at all.

John wondered how this medication would affect him and what else it might do besides lower his blood pressure. He asked if there was anything he could do himself to lower his blood pressure so that he would not have to take medication. The doctor replied that it was probably a good idea to avoid eating too much salt; otherwise, there was nothing to do but take the pills.

Most people in this situation would just do as they were told by their doctor. But John decided he wanted a different opinion and made an appointment to see me. I checked his blood pressure and confirmed that it was higher than it should be, but I also talked with him for a while and learned some interesting things.

He told me that two years ago he had gotten married and that his wife loved rich cooking. As a result, he now ate a good deal more fats and sugar than he had in the past, and during the past two years he had gradually gained about twenty-five pounds. He also told me that during this same period his professional career had rapidly grown more successful. While he was happy with this, he was also very busy and often found himself experiencing considerable stress during the day. Although he had been active in sports for most of his life, he now found that he had little time in his schedule for any physical exercise.

In our brief conversation, he had identified most of the factors typically associated with the development of hypertension. He was overweight, ate a rich diet with too much fat and sugar, did not exercise, and was under increased stress in his life. I explained this to John and told him that he might avoid taking medication if he was willing to try making some changes in his life. I outlined a program that included substantial changes in his diet, a gradual routine of physical exercise, and the regular use of a tape-recorded relaxation exercise, and asked him to come back in six weeks. He was happy to have an alternative to taking medication and assured me that he would follow my advice.

When he returned six weeks later he was enthusiastic about how much better he felt. He had lost several pounds, was jogging regularly, and told me how much more energy he seemed to have. When we checked his blood pressure this time it was normal. We were both very pleased with the result. John had done everything I advised, and I encouraged him to continue with all the changes he had made and return periodically to have his blood pressure checked. There was no longer any need to consider medication at this time.

Admittedly, John was an easy patient. He was young, well-motivated, and basically healthy. Nevertheless, the results were impressive. Compared to the standard treatment of long-term use of drugs that control blood pressure but never actually cure the problem, this was a dramatically successful outcome. Yet there was nothing extraordinary in what I did. There was no new wonder drug, no unusual innovation in treatment, no special skill on my part. All it took was a willingness to look at the patient as an individual and recognize that the signs of illness must be related to that person's life. Any physician prepared to spend a little time and employ a measure of common sense could have accomplished the same thing.

What I do find extraordinary in this story is not my treatment, but the treatment John received from the first doctor. This doctor had become so locked into the routine of diagnosing a specific disease and prescribing a drug for that disease, that he had totally ignored the life situation of his patient. He was not treating John, but his hypertension.

Unfortunately, this is not an unusual situation. Many doctors today would have treated John in the same fashion. But while John was sufficiently independent to seek out another approach, most people would not have been prepared to do this. They would have assumed that if their doctor told them to do something, then it must be right, and they would have taken the prescribed medication. As a result of such medical practice, literally millions of people, not only with hypertension but with many other conditions as well, are routinely put on medications when simple, safe, and natural alternatives for treatment are available.

The Role of Symptoms in Illness

The tendency of modern medicine to treat the illness, rather than the patient, is related to how we define the nature of an illness. What does it mean to say that some-one has high blood pressure? In one sense, high blood pressure is nothing more than a number on a column of mercury. This number represents the pressure developed as blood is pumped through the arteries. We know that chronically high pressures are associated statistically with an increased likelihood of heart disease, strokes, or other serious consequences.

But a reading on a pressure gauge is not an illness. It is an oversimplification to define the problem merely as a number that is too high. While a drug can artificially lower blood pressure, a more useful approach is recogniz-ing the blood pressure reading as one small indicator of the patient's overall condition. To simply lower the blood pressure with a drug is like dealing with a ringing alarm by pulling out the plug. It makes the noise stop, but it does not resolve the condition that caused the alarm to go off.

Although we would surely deal with a ringing alarm more sensibly, this is precisely how millions of people are treated when they are found to have high blood pressure. By defining the problem as the number on the blood pressure cuff, we overlook what is really taking place. I routinely hear announcements on radio and television urging people with high blood pressure to remember their medication, assuring them that if they do so, everything will be fine. These well-intentioned programs may actu-ally do a disservice by encouraging people to believe there is nothing more, aside from taking medication, that needs to be done.

John's high blood pressure was a sign that his lifestyle was beginning to create certain problems in his body and changes were in order. Had he failed to make these changes, his high blood pressure would likely have been followed in the coming years by a succession of other medical problems, whether or not he was taking medication.

Fortunately, he was able to change. The diagnosis of hypertension stimulated him to deal with his condition while it was still easily reversible. It is quite possible that our single brief conversation may have spared him the appearance later in life of a number of serious diseases. Thus, the whole episode had a very positive outcome. An appropriate response to the signs of illness not only resolved the specific problem, but actually led to a state of even better health than he had previously enjoyed.

If John had not had his blood pressure checked, none of this would have happened. He would probably have continued his old pattern of behavior until eventually some more serious illness brought the need for change to his attention. So the blood pressure cuff proved to be a useful device. Like other, far more complex, inventions of medical technology, it allows us to evaluate bodily functions that we could not otherwise detect.

Today we have all sorts of sophisticated devices to observe what is taking place within our bodies. But the information we get from these is only as useful as what we do with it. We publicize programs to check our blood pressure, but what good are they if we just hand out pills to those with high readings? What people really need is to understand the implications of this elevated reading, and to receive guidance from their doctor in recognizing how it is related to what is going on in their lives and what they must do about it.

Understanding the Message of Illness

This discussion could easily have focused on medical problems other than hypertension. Whatever the symptoms of illness may be, they exist for a reason. They are messengers to warn us that, on some level, something is wrong. Their message calls for an appropriate response from the patient in order to resolve the problem that produced the symptom. This response will generally follow a basic pattern. It consists of some *change* in the life of that person so that the symptoms need no longer be present.

This concept of change may be very broadly interpreted. For John, the message was to change to a healthier diet, get more exercise, and learn to manage stress more effectively. Once he did this, there was no longer a need for the message and the symptoms disappeared. Had he not made these changes, other symptoms may have appeared to reinforce the message. And the longer he waited to respond, the more difficult the changes would have been to accomplish. Eventually the continued symptoms might have caused irreversible damage, or perhaps the message would have taken a form so intense that John would have experienced a major heart attack or stroke.

This is one kind of message. The typical American diet and lifestyle are simply not conducive to good health and are responsible for many of today's serious chronic diseases. While this message may take a variety of forms, it is essentially calling attention to the same problem in all those with such illness: changes are needed in how they live and eat if they are to get well.

Mrs. Pratt was a pleasant, overweight woman in her fifties, who had recently developed diabetes. Two years earlier, routine blood tests done during her annual exam had shown abnormally high blood sugar, and she had been started on daily injections of Insulin by her doctor. The Insulin helped control her blood sugar, but it did not change the fact that she had diabetes. It suppressed the most obvious sign of what was going on in her body, but it was not a response to the message conveyed to her by the appearance of diabetes.

While some people with diabetes do require Insulin, this alone does not constitute complete treatment. High blood sugar is not simply a malfunction that can be corrected with a drug; it is an indication of the need for certain changes. Most people who develop diabetes later in life do so because they are overweight, they are not eating a proper diet, and they do not get enough exercise. Thus, when they begin to change these conditions they usually find that their blood sugar goes down. Often it will return completely to normal and all signs of diabetes will disappear.

It is this change in diet, not just a prescription, that is the appropriate response called for by the symptoms. Yet many people with diabetes do not understand this causal connection, and do not realize how closely diabetes is related to factors they can control. Instead, they assume there is nothing to be done but take medication for the rest of their lives. Once Mrs. Pratt realized that she could take responsibility for her own condition, she was able to begin the changes in diet that would enable her to decrease her need for medication.

It is interesting that while hypertension and diabetes are very different diseases, both conditions called for essentially the same response. The changes John made to correct his high blood pressure, and Mrs. Pratt her diabetes, were nearly identical. These two forms of illness manifested in different bodies to convey the same message. Millions of other people are also receiving this message today, each in his or her own way.

However, this is not the only message an illness may contain. Sometimes it is a lot simpler. A cold or sore throat may be telling you nothing more profound than that you need a couple of days rest. When you make this response, the symptoms resolve quickly and that is the end of it. But if you ignore the cold, it may drag on or turn into something more serious.

A smoker with a persistent cough may be getting the message that he must stop smoking to get rid of his cough. Perhaps the runner with a sore knee needs to stop running for a while. The response in these situations is obvious, and if it is not made the symptoms will continue. The smoker may try one cough medicine after another, but he is unlikely to stop coughing until he responds to the real message in the symptom.

If he continues to ignore it, he may do more than keep coughing. Perhaps one day he will even develop cancer. Now it is not enough to just stop smoking; the changes required to get well have become far more profound and may well prove beyond his ability to accomplish. By ignoring the message of a relatively minor symptom, we run the risk that our bodies will eventually resort to a more devastating way of presenting the same message.

Sometimes the necessary response to an illness is not clear. The symptoms may be unpleasant, painful, or frightening, and in the midst of an illness it can be difficult to remember that they are there for a purpose. This is where the physician can really help. His role goes beyond simply removing symptoms; he can help the patient retain the necessary perspective on what he or she is experiencing. When illness of any kind occurs, I find it helpful to ask the question: *What must be changed or done differently so that these symptoms no longer exist?* The answer to this question will contain the key to what must be done.

This is especially useful when the changes required are not made entirely on a physical level. Changing internal emotional states is a more complex undertaking. It may not be immediately apparent how the need for such change is reflected by physical symptoms. A certain amount of mental searching may be required to understand this connection, and it may be up to the doctor to assist in this search and help the patient recognize what is going on in his or her body. This approach is more complicated than swallowing a pill, but also far more rewarding for both doctor and patient.

Discovering the Intention Behind the Symptom

Rachel was a young woman suffering from migraine headaches who went through such a process. She was a professional singer who was very demanding of herself in all aspects of her life. She set high standards for her own performance in anything she did and had a busy, tightly scheduled existence. Approximately every six weeks she would experience a severe migraine headache, with overwhelming pain and nausea, that would often force her to the Emergency Room for a shot of morphine. After a couple of days in bed, her symptoms would subside and she would be fine until the next attack. She had tried various medications and experimented with her diet, but nothing seemed to alter this pattern.

Different theories exist about why people have migraine headaches. In some people, they can apparently be triggered by certain foods, drugs, allergies, the menstrual cycle, or emotional stress. Medical textbooks also describe a particular personality associated with migraines.

The typical patient is a relatively young woman with a tendency toward compulsive or perfectionistic behavior. She is often intelligent, competent, and oriented toward accomplishment in her life. She may spend her days taking care of the children, cleaning the house, pursuing a career, or fulfilling whatever set of individual responsibilities she has assumed. She will usually take on more than she can comfortably handle, so that she is always busy with something. No matter how hard she tries, she can never quite get everything done well enough for her own exacting standards. The house never seems clean enough, or the children never receive all the attention they need, or some other responsibility is inevitably neglected in her closely scheduled day.

Eventually, the pressure builds to a point where it finally bursts out, both physically and symbolically, in the form of a migraine headache. This effectively breaks the cycle. The headaches are generally incapacitating, and force her to spend a day or two doing nothing but lying in bed in a dark room. In this very dramatic fashion, the pressure is at last released, and for a short time she can abandon her responsibilities. However, once the headache is over, the same pattern resumes and the pressure gradually begins to build again. This continues until it is once again interrupted by the next headache. This may happen in a week or several weeks, or months may go by between headaches, depending on the individual and what is happening in her life.

This is a composite picture of many people with migraine headaches. Obviously it fits some better than others, but for the most part I have found it surprisingly accurate. Certainly it applied very well to Rachel. When approached as a disease that she happened to have, her migraines were an unpleasant occurrence to be suppressed as much as possible with whatever drugs would do the job. But when seen in the context of her life situation, the headaches took on a different meaning. It was apparent that there was a reason for their existence.

Rachel had adopted a way of living that was too exhausting to sustain. Periodically she required a break from this routine, but the only way she could allow this was by having a headache. This was the message, and in providing this message, the headaches served an important purpose in her life.

Rachel needed her headaches. Without them there would be no opportunity to escape the pressures of daily existence. Why she chose migraines to accomplish this rather than some other symptom is another question. Perhaps she had some biochemical predisposition toward this condition, but this is only a partial explanation. Her headaches could only be fully understood in the context of what was happening in her life.

Various drugs may partially relieve migraines, but drugs will rarely eliminate them entirely. This is not surprising. If headaches are serving a real purpose for the patient, such as providing the only means of relief from daily pressures, it will be difficult to make them disappear. If they should be suppressed completely, the body will simply find another avenue for conveying its message to the individual.

One woman's case illustrated very well how this can happen. For years this woman had suffered from migraine headaches, and her doctor had tried one drug after another without success. Then one day he tried a new drug that really seemed to work. Several months went by without a migraine and she was delighted with the result. But eventually she noticed that a new symptom had appeared.

She began to experience severe muscle spasms in her neck, at times so incapacitating that she would spend a day or two in bed. These neck pains now served the same purpose her migraines had in the past. She appeared to have exchanged one symptom for the other, although she herself was unaware of any connection between them. She had come to me for treatment of her neck pain, but she did not need more symptomatic relief. Treating her neck would probably not help any more than getting rid of her migraines, unless she was able to respond to the *cause* of these symptoms. As with Rachel, her headaches and neck pain gave her a way to get some badly needed rest.

If the symptoms of illness fulfill a real purpose, then they can only be removed if this purpose is addressed. It is important to realize that this purpose is not a bad one, and that symptoms are not necessarily something negative to be avoided. In a sense, the intention behind the symptom of a headache can be good. It allows the opportunity for rest and the release of accumulated tension. The problem is not the intention, but the unpleasant way in which it is accomplished.

A migraine headache is not the only way, and certainly not the best way, to take a rest. For real healing to take place, what is needed is another, more constructive, way to accomplish what the headaches are now doing. What Rachel required was a change in life patterns that would allow her to rest without first having to develop a headache. Developing such an alternative pattern is often an essential part of dealing with any illness.

When I began to see Rachel, I agreed to continue her pain medication, in case of a really severe headache. I also began a course of acupuncture, which is often an effective treatment for migraines. I suspect acupuncture works by allowing a release of tension on some level in the body, so that it is less likely to build up to the point of precipitating a headache.

Rachel was also treated with massage and began an exercise program, both of which may have a similar tension-releasing effect. As treatment continued, her headaches occurred less often, but they did not go away entirely. Something more was needed to achieve this result. We continued to work on understanding why her headaches occurred when they did, and what changes they were telling her to make.

This was not easy for her, but eventually she reached a point where her headaches no longer felt like a major interference in her life. There was a change in her attitude toward them. She now saw the headaches not as something terrible that happened to her, but as a kind of feedback from her body about what she was doing.

While her occasional headaches were still unpleasant, she could accept one as a signal to look at what could have precipitated it. Her symptoms were not completely gone, but she no longer felt no control over the situation.

Symptoms as Catalyst for Change

The message of a particular symptom is not necessarily the same for everyone. Sally was a patient whose headaches served a somewhat different purpose. She was a dark-haired, slender woman of twenty-five, who spoke softly and seemed shy and ill at ease in conversation. Her headaches were not migraines, but were of the muscle tension variety, beginning at the base of the skull and temples and progressing to a throbbing pain across her entire head. These headaches had become increasingly frequent, until Sally often found herself swallowing aspirin tablets throughout the day. At last she decided something must be done and made an appointment to see a doctor.

Although she may not have expressed herself in these words, she was essentially saying two things to the doctor: "I am worried by these headaches. Tell me if there is anything seriously wrong with me," and "I don't like these headaches. Please do something to make them go away." Regardless of the particular symptoms, these are typically the two fundamental concerns any patient brings to a doctor: tell me what is wrong with me and make it go away.

Doctors are usually good at answering the first request, at least on the physical level. Her doctor ordered every possible test to investigate her headaches, including an EEG and a CT-scan of her head, and in the end informed her that all results were normal. He advised her that there was "nothing wrong with her" and that her headaches were simply due to tension.

Although this was reassuring in a way, it did not tell her how to make the headaches go away. For this, the doctor was considerably less helpful. All he had to offer was a prescription for some stronger pain pills than the aspirin she was already taking.

Having gone through the time, expense, and discomfort of a full medical work-up, Sally was frustrated with the result. Clearly there was *something* wrong, but she did not know what else to do. Her story is typical of many people's experience with our medical system. They receive an elaborate evaluation, but in the end they may not get a meaningful answer about what is troubling them.

This is because doctors often devote their time to looking for these answers in the wrong places. While it is certainly important to identify the rare patient with a brain tumor or some other unusual abnormality that may be causing headaches, it is not necessary to order a five-hundred-dollar CT-scan on every person who complains of headaches. It is far more likely the doctor will learn something about why a person has headaches by talking with him for a while, rather than by studying an X-ray of his head. Modern medicine has wonderful machines that allow us to look inside of people's heads, but this is not necessarily where we will find the answers to their medical problems. Instead, we need to look inside their lives and feelings, which, in its own way, can be a more complex undertaking.

In order to accomplish this with Sally, I asked her to begin keeping a journal of when her headaches occurred. From this journal a simple and consistent pattern emerged. Whenever she was in an uncomfortable situation she would get a headache. And for Sally it appeared that many situations were uncomfortable, especially when other people were involved. It was difficult for her to express her feelings and frequently she found herself going along with what other people wanted. In order to avoid such situations or say no to other people, she had discovered that a headache could provide an effective, socially acceptable solution.

This was not a conscious choice on her part. Rather, it was a successful form of behavior her body had learned in order to get out of difficult situations. As with Rachel, the woman with migraines, Sally's headaches were basically serving a constructive purpose. The problem again was not *what* the symptoms were attempting to accomplish, but *how* this was being done. Once she was aware of the pattern of her headaches, she could begin to learn a less unpleasant way of coping with difficult situations.

As she examined what took place each time she developed a headache, Sally learned more about her own behavior. She began to develop a sense of what she wanted in different situations, and gradually her behavior changed. As this happened, her headaches grew less frequent and severe. She had moved from wanting someone else to make her headaches go away, to understanding why she had headaches and what she herself needed to do differently.

This was a very significant step. As she was able to do this, not only did her headaches decrease, but she felt generally more satisfied with herself than she had before. The presence of the symptom and the process of understanding what it meant had actually served as a stimulus to personal growth for her. This positive outcome can often be achieved when we are able to make a genuinely constructive response not only to headaches, but to any physical symptom that is serving a similar purpose.

4

Symptoms as Symbol

Interpreting the Message

Often in working with patients, my role as a doctor has been not only to *treat* symptoms, although this is sometimes necessary, but also to help *interpret their meaning*. This is an endlessly fascinating aspect of medical practice. It entails recognizing the remarkably symbolic nature that illness sometimes assumes.

For example, a person or situation we do not like may be referred to as a "headache." This is not a random choice of words. It comes from a recognition that these are the sorts of things that produce the physical symptom of a headache. For Sally, the young woman in the previous chapter, certain aspects of life were quite literally a headache. And acknowledging this rather obvious symbolism was important for understanding what had to be done for her.

An unpleasant person or situation may also be described as a "pain in the neck," or, a bit more crudely, as a "pain in the ass." Interestingly, neck pain or low back pain are also common reactions to stressful or unpleasant situations. The fundamental cause of neck pain will often turn out to be some situation in a person's life that he finds a "pain in the neck." While the symbolic nature of these examples seems obvious, often it is not at all obvious to the person actually experiencing the symptom. Someone may search for a variety of explanations to account for the pain, when, to an outside observer, the relationship between his pain and some situation in his life is immediately apparent.

It is surprising how often this connection is ignored in medical practice. You do not have to go to medical school to know that stressful life situations can be a "pain in the ass." But among patients with low back pain, the role of stress in creating their symptoms may receive little attention. Medical care of low back pain tends to focus on the purely physical aspect of the problem, but often there is more involved.

Doctors and Low Back Pain

Physicians who regularly see patients with low back pain often observe that many of these patients are also depressed. The explanation could simply be that these people are depressed because they are in pain, but it is interesting to look at it from the other direction. Perhaps they are experiencing pain *because* they are depressed. This makes for another situation entirely. Or maybe the pain and depression are not really related as cause and effect, but as different expressions of the same underlying state. Perhaps the best way to view these symptoms is as the physical and emotional sides of what is being experienced by the whole person.

Why is low back pain such a common complaint? Why the low back rather than some other part of the body? Part of the explanation may be purely mechanical. The low back is especially vulnerable to strain among a population of sedentary, often overweight, people who rarely engage in vigorous physical activity. As a result of this inactivity, the muscles of the low back and abdomen often are not well developed and are easily strained beyond their capacity.

One possible consequence of back strain is a diagnosis of "herniated disc," a condition in which one of the vertebral discs—pieces of tough, fibrous material in the shape of a disc that lie between and cushion each of the vertebrae of the spine—becomes pushed from its normal position between the vertebrae. This displaced disc can produce pressure on nearby nerves as they leave the spine, causing pain along the course of the involved nerves, as well as weakness or loss of sensation in parts of the legs.

Initial treatment of a herniated disc is usually bed rest, but if this does not produce noticeable improvement, then the next step is surgery. If a displaced disc is producing pressure on nerves, then the solution of modern medicine is to cut away a portion of the disc that is creating the pressure. This type of surgery is called a laminectomy, and it has become a routine procedure for millions of people with low back pain.

Sometimes, serious nerve compression is present, and a laminectomy is clearly needed to prevent permanent damage. But many times the indications for this surgery are more open to question. Typically, a patient will complain of back pain, his X-rays indicate some disc displacement, and the doctor decides to operate. The assumption is that the disc is the sole cause of the problem, but this explanation may be too simple.

Unfortunately, cutting away the disc does not always solve the problem. A significant number of people do not get relief from back surgery, or the pain recurs soon after the operation. This may be the beginning of an endless round of back problems. If the patient continues to complain of pain, the eventual solution may be another operation, perhaps on a different disc. Some people have two, three, or even more operations on their back, and still have pain.

It is very sad to find someone in this situation. I have seen people whose lower backs are literally criss-crossed with surgical scars and the normal anatomy totally destroyed, yet still complaining of pain. Whatever their condition may have been before surgery, they certainly do not have a normal back now and never will again, and it is difficult to do anything to free them from pain. It is a delicate business to tamper with the structures of the spine, and I have seen enough people with poor results of low back surgery to be wary of this procedure.

I suspect that many laminectomies performed today are unnecessary. Nevertheless, this operation remains popular because it is a natural conclusion of the current medical perspective on the problem. The idea that back pain is produced solely by the mechanical pressure of a protruding disc upon adjacent nerves has an appealing simplicity, but the reality may be more complex. The low back is not static; like the rest of the body, it is in a process of constant adjustment, so that displacement of a disc is not necessarily a completely unchangeable condition.

It is also interesting to consider more esoteric explanations of how the low back can become a focus of pain. In Eastern systems of medicine, the energy centers of the body corresponding to the more basic biological functions are said to exist in the region of the lower spine. This part of the body, both physically, in terms of major nerve centers, and metaphysically, in terms of energy centers, corresponds to bodily functions involving physical survival, elimination, and sexuality. From this perspective, pain and tension in the lower back could be the physical representation of a problem in this aspect of a person's life.

Choosing Health or Illness

Martha was a young woman who had complained of low back pain for almost a year when I first saw her. She had already been to two or three other doctors with no help. There were no objective signs of nerve damage, only the presence of pain, and we were left with the vague diagnosis of "sciatica" or "low back syndrome." Recently her pain had become worse, and because medications and physical therapy had not really helped, she was interested in trying acupuncture.

I worked with Martha for about four months. During this time, she was treated not only with acupuncture, but with massage, an exercise program, and another course of physical therapy. Nothing helped for any length of time. Occasionally she improved slightly for a while, but then the pain would return again, as bad as before. She consulted a new orthopedic surgeon, but he had nothing further to offer. She even obtained a leave from her job as a secretary to give her back a complete rest, but this made no difference either.

Martha was a robust-looking woman whose most striking feature was her long blonde hair. She had a powerful, muscular body, and the various therapists who had worked with her were at first optimistic that she would make a good recovery. After treatment, they were always puzzled as to why she did not get better. She was intelligent and well spoken, and she assured us there were no problems in her life. She liked her husband, she liked her job, she liked her home; she was quite happy, except for her back pain. If only it would go away, everything would be fine.

I am always a little suspicious when someone assures me so adamantly that everything, except a particular symptom, is fine. Often it turns out that the symptom is there because everything is *not* fine, on some level. But whenever I raised the possibility of an emotional aspect to her symptoms, she would not even consider the idea.

As far as she was concerned, there was something physically wrong with her back, and nobody had been able to come up with the right treatment yet. For Martha, discussion of anything else was irrelevant. Still, I sensed a discordant note. Somehow she did not seem as happy as she claimed to be.

Eventually it became clear that what we were doing was not going to help her. On one of her final visits, we talked about what had been happening in her life when the pain first appeared, and she related an incident she had never mentioned before. About a year ago, she discovered her husband had had an affair with another woman. She had been very angry and hurt, but she and her husband had talked it over and ostensibly resolved what had happened.

On the surface, she had put the whole episode behind her and the marriage was now going smoothly. But it was apparent that she still carried a great deal of anger that had never been fully expressed. She also felt insecure about her marriage, and secretly wondered if the same thing might happen again, though she never spoke of this to her husband.

It was obviously difficult for her to talk about all of this, and I wondered whether these powerful but unexpressed feelings of anger, resentment, and insecurity were finding physical expression in her continued back pain. Certainly, her persistent tension about the affair was related to her sense of basic security and her sexuality. If this were the case, she might need to express and resolve these feelings more fully before her back pain could be eliminated. This might explain why this seemingly robust young woman was not making progress with her back problem, no matter what treatment we tried.

I approached this idea carefully, but without success. Martha made it quite clear that she was not interested in pursuing the problem on this level, and quickly brought the conversation back to a more neutral topic. Perhaps it was actually easier for her to deal with continued back pain than to bring her feelings into conscious consideration.

I saw Martha once more after this. She told me she had applied for disability status in order to remain off work indefinitely. She also had an appointment with a new orthopedist to discuss injections in her low back as treatment. I was sorry to see her move in this direction. I felt she was on a path, taken by many others before her, toward becoming a person with a life long back problem.

I saw ahead of her an endless round of visits to the doctor, X-rays, consultations with specialists, and perhaps, eventually, even surgery, if she complained of the pain long enough. She would follow this course because she focused on the symptom of pain itself, rather than on the meaning behind it. What she really needed was to confront her emotional pain and eventually pass through it, rather than to hold it indefinitely in the physical form of low back pain.

Fortunately, not all patients with low back pain experience such an unhappy outcome. Tom was an architect in his forties who exercised regularly and was in good physical condition. But a week after doing some carpentry work, he suddenly developed pain in his low back that radiated down one leg. He was quite uncomfortable, and had come to see about the possibility of acupuncture treatment. I agreed to treat him and then we talked for a while about what had been happening in his life.

For some time he had been having problems with his marriage. Recently, his wife had become involved with another man, and two days before the onset of his back pain, she had moved out of the house. He had also been going through a personal crisis regarding his work. After much internal struggle, he had decided to abandon the architectural profession he had followed for most of his life, although he was unsure of what he would do instead.

In a very short span of time, the basic security of his life, which had for years been built upon his home, his marriage, and his work, had collapsed. He had also been wounded sexually by his wife leaving him for another man, and it was clearly painful for him to talk about this. His speech and behavior were subdued and conveyed a sense of depression.

It would be foolish to treat his low back pain without considering the context in which it had occurred. While there was undoubtedly a mechanical aspect to the pain, it was also clearly related to what was going on in his life. Anybody experiencing such a major personal crisis is likely to develop some physical symptom. For Tom, low back pain seemed to be an appropriate expression of his particular situation.

Fortunately, he did not become preoccupied with the purely physical aspect of his symptoms. He accepted the connection between the back pain and what was happening in his life. He realized that he had been dissatisfied with his marriage and his work, and that the changes now happening, although painful, could eventually lead his life in a positive direction.

He could even see that the back pain itself was serving a certain purpose. Initially, he had responded to the upheaval in his life with almost frantic activity in order to keep himself occupied. Now he could see that he needed to simply rest and do nothing as he assimilated and processed what had happened. This was accomplished effectively by his back pain, which precluded any activity. Once he accepted this, he found the enforced rest a great relief.

Without coming to terms with his life situation, the outcome for Tom might have been very painful and difficult. Fortunately, he was able to understand the reason for his back pain and respond to it appropriately. With the help of acupuncture treatment and a chance to talk a little about what he was experiencing, Tom made a prompt and complete recovery.

Emotions and Physical Symptoms

Symptoms other than pain may also have a symbolic meaning that can point the way to appropriate treatment. Yet, physicians often become so caught up in the mechanics of diagnosis and treatment that they pay no attention to this very useful information.

Denise was an attractive, well-groomed woman of about thirty, with the somewhat unusual complaint of numbness and tingling in her arms, which she had had for the past two years. She would experience this sensation at various times, especially during the night, when she would sometimes awaken with the feeling that her arms were "asleep." She had consulted a number of different doctors but had never received a clear diagnosis. When the episodes of numbness became more frequent, she was referred to a University medical center for evaluation. Though the doctors there had performed extensive tests, they were still puzzled and were now contemplating some surgical procedure designed to relieve pressure on the nerves to her arms.

My first impression of Denise as she entered my office was one of sadness. Her face, and especially her eyes, gave a strong sense of someone who was frightened and unhappy. As she walked across the room, I noticed the obvious tension in her movements; this tension became even more apparent when I examined her. Her neck and shoulders were extremely tight and tender, and, in particular, the muscles across the tops of her shoulders were as hard as rocks.

As we talked, Denise told me she had left her husband six months ago and was still not reconciled to the separation. She was torn between her desire to escape the difficulties of her marriage and her urge to return home and try again. This prolonged internal conflict had exhausted her. She felt she was in a situation where no choice seemed right, and the strain was reflected in her physical body.

I was convinced that her symptoms were related to this conflict. Their pattern did not fit any known neurological disorder, and none of her doctors had found any specific abnormality. It seemed most likely that chronic stress had created an unusual tension in her neck and shoulder muscles, which, in turn, was producing pressure on the nerve trunks to the arms.

This explanation made a lot of sense to her, although, for Denise, the idea of a connection between her symptoms and her emotional state was quite new. None of the many doctors she had seen had so much as mentioned this possibility. Their concerns had been focused on diagnosing some unusual neurological condition and determining whether or not she might be helped with surgery.

However, surgery seemed to be the last thing she needed. I sent for her records from the University to see what the doctors there were thinking. A few days later, a thick envelope arrived with extensive laboratory records and reports of consultations with three different neurologists. They had been very thorough. Each report ran to several pages, and I was impressed by how carefully she had been examined. Each specialist described in detail the results of his examination, analyzed the laboratory tests, and discussed at length the possible diagnosis. Yet in all these pages, not one doctor had devoted a single word to her emotional state or life circumstances, let alone considered whether these might have some relation to her symptoms.

I cannot believe this is because the doctors were unaware of Denise's circumstances. From the moment she entered my office I was struck by the sadness in her eyes. On one occasion, even my receptionist commented on how unhappy Denise seemed. She felt no professional obligation to ignore her natural response to another human being. After talking with Denise for a while, she could probably have told more about what was really wrong with her than all the medical specialists using thousands of dollars of lab work to diagnose her illness. Somehow her doctors had separated their human perception from what was relevant to their professional role. Unfortunately, this had prevented them from recognizing the most important information for understanding the patient.

In any event, I was relieved to learn that the consultants had found no clear indication for surgery and had nothing further to propose. I continued to see Denise for a while, but various treatments provided her only modest improvement. She remained in the same ambivalent state about her marriage, and I suspected her symptoms might continue until this was somehow resolved.

But now at least she could understand the source of the numbness and its connection to her emotional life. This was a considerable relief for her, as she no longer had to spend her energy consulting different doctors and worrying about what strange disease she might have. Although she still had the symptoms, she could devote herself to dealing with the issues in her life that really needed attention.

For Denise, numbness in her arms was the symbolic expression of withdrawal from another person she still loved. Jane was a patient who expressed a similar feeling through a somewhat different, but symbolically equivalent, symptom. She had Raynaud's disease, a circulatory disturbance involving temporary loss of blood flow to one or more fingers. When this occurs, the affected fingers will turn white, cold, and numb for several minutes or even hours. The cause is not well understood, but episodes of Raynaud's disease are typically precipitated by exposure to cold, and may also be related to emotional stress.

For years, Jane had experienced only occasional mild symptoms. Shortly after leaving her husband, however, these had abruptly become much worse. One of her fingers had become permanently numb and cold, and actually developed an ulcer at the tip due to continued loss of circulation. Like Denise, she was in a situation of withdrawing from a person she had loved, and for her, the symbolic equivalent was the withdrawal of circulation from her hands.

Jane was treated with various drugs intended to improve circulation by another physician specializing in such problems. At the same time, I also worked with her on recognizing how her physical symptoms were related to what she was feeling. With this combined therapy, she eventually made a full recovery. She was able to realize that the ulcer on her finger had not appeared with no reason, but was connected to her emotional state. This was a less frightening prospect. It allowed her to feel that she could regain some control over what was taking place in her body. It also gave her a perspective for dealing with future episodes of her disease, not as something unpleasant, but as feedback on her own feelings.

If doctor and patient are open to looking for the symbolic connection between physical symptoms and the patient's life situation, it is remarkable how often such a connection is there to be found. Recognizing this connection not only adds a new dimension to the symptoms, but also sheds light on what must be done about them.

It is no coincidence that most of the above examples have involved difficulties in close relationships. This is one of the most frequent precipitating factors for physical illness, and it is important for anyone with a troublesome physical symptom to recognize when this may be happening in his or her life. It is necessary for a doctor to pay serious attention to this aspect of his patient's life. Events in close personal relationships cannot be dismissed as a nonmedical concern, as so often happens; indeed, they may be the only way to fully appreciate the meaning behind the physical symptoms.

Symptoms are the language of the body. Often they are the language of the emotions or of the unconscious part of ourselves that is given physical expression. Psychologist Carl Jung wrote that illness could be thought of as the consequence of a separation and loss of communication between the conscious and unconscious parts of the self, and that therapy consists of somehow restoring this communication. This may apply not only to psychological illness, but to illness that takes a physical form, as well. If we pay attention to symptoms, we may discover that their message is an attempt by the body to restore a connection between different parts of the whole person.

However, the message may not be easy to hear or to accept. If it were easy, it would not need to assume the form of illness to demand our attention. Some who are ill never respond to this message. The necessary changes required appear too difficult, or too painful, and it seems preferable to continue to be sick. Perhaps Martha, for example, the woman with low back pain, found it easier to accept continued physical pain in her back than to confront the emotional pain beneath it. This is not a conscious choice, but it is nevertheless a real one.

Sometimes symptoms become so severe it is necessary to do something to relieve them. But if this is the doctor's sole purpose, it limits medical practice to only a part of what it can really accomplish. It is also up to the doctor to help his patient understand the connection between symptoms and events happening in his life, and at least point in the right direction for appropriate change. Beyond this, it becomes the responsibility of the patient to decide what he is prepared to do. However, he at least deserves the opportunity to realize that this choice exists, and to make it himself.

Sometimes, just the realization that a medical problem exists for a comprehensible reason can be therapeutic in itself. The patient no longer feels entirely at the mercy of some mysterious ailment; he can at least understand why it is present and what must be done to deal with it, even if the actual healing process may take some time. Thus, instead of being an unexplained, random intrusion into the normal routine, illness becomes something that has a meaning in the context of our lives.

When we understand this meaning, we can even see that illness may have a positive side. After an illness has run its course, and a successful response has been made, you can sometimes look back on the experience and see that, if you had not become sick, you would never have learned certain things, or done certain things, or made certain changes that now have a positive influence on the future direction of your life. If we learn to listen carefully to our bodies, we will often find that they tell us just what we need to know.

5

Muscles, Emotions, and Illness

The Muscular Structure

The physical body commonly reflects emotional stress through the muscular system. Conditions of abnormal muscle tension or spasm often occur and produce symptoms that prompt a visit to the doctor. However, these conditions are frequently not recognized for what they really are. This is because doctors tend to overlook the importance of the state of the muscular system in evaluating health. It would be unthinkable for a doctor to perform a general examination without listening to the patient's heart and lungs, or palpating his abdominal organs, but he might easily omit all examination of the muscles and connective tissues.

It is almost as though we think of bones and muscles as little more than a static framework for containing the organs, nerves, blood vessels, and other essential structures of life. But muscles, too, are "alive," and the state of the body's muscular structure can play a far greater role in illness than is often appreciated.

Conditions of chronic pain that originates in the muscular system are referred to by a variety of names. We call them "myofascial pain syndromes" or "fibrositis" or "fibromyalgia," to mention a few of the cumbersome names given such conditions. This confusion of terms reflects the fact that these conditions are not clearly understood in medical practice today. However, all the names describe the same basic process: an abnormal state of the muscles and connective tissue in some part of the body that produces a particular pattern of pain.

Typically, these conditions involve a focus of pain at one or more specific points in the muscle. These points are referred to as "trigger points." They are extremely tender to the touch, and sometimes a small, hard knot can be felt in the muscle at the point of greatest tenderness. The diagnosis of a trigger point is established when pressure on the point precisely reproduces the pain being experienced.

Trigger points can occur anywhere in the body, but certain places are especially common. Very often, the muscles of the neck, shoulders, and upper back are involved. The trapezius muscle—the large, fan-shaped muscle that stretches from the base of the skull across the top of the shoulder—is probably the most common source of pain symptoms that I encounter.

Several different trigger points can be found within this muscle. One of the most characteristic is located midway across the top of the shoulder in the thickest part of the muscle. Often a knot can be felt here as well. Pressure at this point will produce a typical pattern of referred pain along the side of the neck, around the ear, and into the temple or base of the skull.

One interesting study examined a large group of patients who described this pattern of pain. It was found that all of them had a trigger point in the identical location in the trapezius muscle. The study went on to show that they could be treated by injecting a local anaesthetic directly into the muscle at the trigger point. This would give prompt relief of pain which might even continue after the anaesthetic had worn off. Occasionally, the pain relief would be long-lasting and possibly even permanent.

What is even more interesting, however, is that simply inserting a needle into the same point without injecting anything may have a similar result. This is sometimes called "dry needling," and its effectiveness will not be mysterious for anyone familiar with acupuncture. It turns out that the point in the trapezius muscle, like most trigger points, is also an acupuncture point. Its anatomical location is identical with a frequently used acupuncture point, and injection or dry needling at this point is actually acupuncture called by a different name.

I rarely examine anyone who does not have at least a little tightness in the trapezius and associated neck muscles, and for many people it is a familiar area of discomfort. However, it is not always realized that tension in these muscles can produce not only local pain, but a variety of other symptoms as well. These include dizziness, ringing in the ears, nausea, pain radiating down the arm, and, particularly, headaches. I have seen patients undergo elaborate medical investigation of headaches or dizziness, when a simple examination of their muscles would have revealed the source of the problem immediately.

An Explanation for Headaches

Mark was a young man who had complained of severe headaches for months. They would begin at the base of his skull and sometimes were associated with light-headedness or actual dizziness. Mark had seen several doctors, including a neurologist and an ear, nose, and throat specialist, and had undergone a variety of laboratory tests. All of these tests were normal; nevertheless, his symptoms persisted.

When I examined Mark, I found tremendous tightness in the muscles along both sides of his neck and in his shoulders. The trapezius muscles were particularly tender, and when I pressed on the most sensitive spot in the center of the muscle, he immediately felt a wave of dizziness and nausea. I felt the diagnosis was obvious. Any of his other doctors could have made this diagnosis without elaborate tests, had they simply examined the condition of his muscles.

Chronic muscle tension is often a reponse to stress, and there was a lot going on in Mark's life that could have been creating this stress. He worked as an accountant for a large corporation, but did not get along with his supervisor. The supervisor wanted to fire him, but company regulations made this difficult without a good reason. However, while the supervisor could not find a way to actually fire Mark, he could make the job very uncomfortable for him. It had reached a point where Mark dreaded going to work in the morning, and by the end of the day his neck and shoulders were a mass of knots.

Mark often dealt with the situation by escaping into alcohol or marijuana as soon as he got home. He was beginning to worry that these habits were getting out of control. He was also worried about why he felt dizzy so much, and whether this indicated there was something seriously wrong with him. The more he worried, the more stressful the entire situation became, and the more stressful things were, the worse his neck became. By the time I saw Mark, he was caught in this negative spiral, and the various aspects of his problem were all reinforcing each other.

Probably the most helpful thing I was able to do was explain that his symptoms were not a sign of some mysterious disease, but the result of simple muscle tension. I treated Mark with a course of acupuncture, which provided a lot of relief. As he began to feel better, he was able to reduce his use of alcohol and marijuana. His symptoms did not go away entirely, but they were no longer out of control. He was at least able to understand what was going on in his body.

Mark's difficulty in getting clear diagnosis and treatment from his doctors was not unusual. Many people with this type of condition have a similar experience. Typically, they are treated with pain pills, tranquilizers, antidepressants, or other drugs that, at best, give only temporary relief. Sometimes they are told there is nothing wrong with them, because no abnormality appears on lab tests or X-rays. Even worse, they may be misdiagnosed as having some problem that does not really exist.

Making the Correct Diagnosis

A twenty-five-year-old woman I saw who was suffering from pain in her shoulder and arm was told by another doctor that she had "rheumatoid arthritis." This diagnosis of what can be a serious and often crippling disease had caused this young woman a great deal of anxiety. Fortunately, it was totally incorrect. There was no basis for a diagnosis of rheumatoid arthritis, and her symptoms were, in fact, not related to arthritis of any kind. This was yet another case of muscle tension produced by emotional stress, and the condition responded well to treatment that dealt with this tension. Not only did she find relief from her pain, she was also enormously relieved to learn it had nothing to do with rheumatoid arthritis.

Although this was an extreme example of misdiagnosis, the term "arthritis" tends to be applied very loosely to many forms of muscle or joint pain. It has become a catch-all term for the daily aches and pains that parade through the doctor's office in the course of a day. The problem with this kind of diagnosis is that it leads to inappropriate treatment. An incorrect diagnosis of arthritis may mean people will be given drugs that are unnecessary, ineffective for treating what is actually wrong with them, and sometimes even dangerous. It also leads them to believe they are suffering from a life-long condition, when, in fact, what they are experiencing may be entirely reversible.

The possibility of misdiagnosis is even more likely when problems originating in muscles lead not to pain, but to more unusual symptoms. Mrs. Robbins was a woman in her late forties who experienced the mysterious and troublesome symptom of severe vertigo when moving her head to certain positions. She was unable to lie on her right side without experiencing overwhelming sensations of dizziness and nausea, and would be awakened out of a sound sleep by intense whirling sensations if she inadvertently turned the wrong way.

After a full medical evaluation, including an array of sophisticated neurological tests, she had been given a diagnosis of "benign positional vertigo." However, this diagnosis did no more than provide a descriptive name for her symptoms, and did not suggest what she might do about them. She had tried the usual drugs with no result, and had decided to find out if acupuncture might help.

As I listened to her story, I was not sure at first if I would be able to do anything. However, when it came time to examine her, I made some interesting observations. Certain movements of her head and eyes would consistently elicit strong sensations of vertigo, something that had been noted by her neurologists. But the same sensations could also be produced by pressure on certain acupuncture points in the back of her neck. This suggested a way to approach the problem, and I was encouraged to begin a course of acupuncture treatment.

Mrs. Robbins responded well from the start. Almost immediately she noticed a decrease in her symptoms and began to sleep better at night. Soon she was even able to turn on her right side without being awakened by vertigo. She continued to make good progress, and before long her dizziness had almost vanished.

The most likely explanation was that her dizziness had been an unusual symptom of myofascial tension in the neck. I suspect similar conditions may be involved in other cases of unexplained vertigo. Yet, even though medical textbooks list far more obscure causes of vertigo, you will rarely find this possibility discussed at any length.

TMJ Syndrome

Perhaps the most overlooked and misdiagnosed of all myofascial conditions is temporomandibular joint (TMJ) syndrome. It involves pain at the temporomandibular joint, where the mandible, or lower jaw bone, connects to the skull, the place just in front of the ear that moves as you chew.

TMJ syndrome falls somewhere between the province of physicians and that of dentists, and often is not fully understood by either. There is much difference of opinion about what causes this problem to begin. Sometimes it can be traced to dental work or an injury to the jaw, and typically there is improper occlusion of the teeth.

Regardless of the initial cause, TMJ syndrome is invariably characterized by tension and spasm of the jaw muscles. This may be on one side only, but more often occurs on both. Like other forms of muscle tension, spasm of the jaw muscles is related to stress, usually expressed by clenching the jaws, often unconsciously, or repeatedly grinding the teeth. These habits are especially common during sleep, and the person may be entirely unaware of what he or she is doing. Eventually the jaw joints become painful, and muscle spasm may be so severe that it is difficult to open the mouth.

TMJ syndrome can also cause pain throughout the head, and is commonly experienced as headache, toothache, earache, or other complaints. Most people who awaken in the morning with headaches are suffering from TMJ syndrome produced by unconscious clenching of the jaw muscles during sleep. Some grind their teeth so extensively that the tooth surfaces become severely worn down. This symptom will be apparent to a doctor or dentist who examines the patient, and its appearance can help diagnose a TMJ problem.

Although TMJ syndrome has only recently become well known, it is surprisingly common, especially among young women. It is easy to diagnose, but many doctors still do not think of it as a possible cause of symptoms they observe. Thus, people with TMJ syndrome may make the rounds of dentists and medical specialists to find an explanation for their symptoms.

I have seen such patients undergo extensive X-rays and laboratory tests to diagnose their problem, without ever finding the real cause. Others have been incorrectly diagnosed as having ear infections and treated with antibiotics, sometimes repeatedly, and always, of course, without success. Still others have had teeth pulled in a futile attempt to relieve their pain, while the true source of their trouble was located in the jaw muscles.

I recall one man with chronic headaches who had seen an unusual number of doctors. Finally one specialist had told him his headaches were related to a sinus problem, and suggested a major surgical procedure on his sinuses to correct this. Out of desperation to find anything that could help, he was considering this surgery, although with much reluctance.

Upon examination, it was immediately apparent that his headaches were caused by TMJ syndrome. This had never been mentioned by anyone he had seen, and the explanation was a revelation to him. As is often the case, the mere understanding of what was going on was an important step toward being able to resolve the problem. He had been unaware of tension in his jaw muscles, but now that he recognized it, he could try to correct it. I saw him only once but I heard several weeks later that he was making progress and had abandoned any thought of surgery.

As with most difficult medical problems, a great variety of treatments for TMJ syndrome is available. The one you get will usually depend on who you see. TMJ problems are often treated by dentists, most of whom tend to concentrate their attention on how the teeth meet. They work from the premise that improper occlusion of the teeth is the primary cause of the problem, and that pain and muscle spasm develop secondary to this condition. They conclude that if they can correct how the teeth meet, then they can correct the whole problem.

Dentists often try to accomplish this by constructing a small plastic splint to fit between the upper and lower teeth. Its purpose is to correct the bite, and also to protect the tooth surfaces from further wear by grinding. It is usually worn throughout the night and sometimes during the day as well.

While these splints will prevent continued damage to the teeth, this approach to treatment has certain limitations. In my own experience, most TMJ problems seem more complicated than an incorrect bite. In many cases, it seems to be the chronic spasm of the jaw muscles that distorts normal alignment of the teeth, rather than the other way around. And while adjustment of the bite may help, it will not lead to permanent change as long as the muscles remain in spasm. If tension in the jaw muscles is created by emotional stress, then successful treatment may have to address this underlying cause and do something to enable these muscles to relax.

Whether they involve the jaw or some other part of the body, myofascial pain problems often represent unreleased tension in the body, which has been created by strong emotions that, for some reason, are not adequately expressed. Feelings of anger, fear, or frustration can show up in the body as tight, painful muscles. For example, when you hold back angry words, we sometimes say that "you bite your tongue." An obvious symbolic expression of this would be to clench the muscles of your jaw. If this happens regularly, it would not be surprising to observe the appearance of TMJ syndrome.

One woman with a severe and long-standing TMJ problem told me she would never allow herself to raise her voice or express anger toward her husband or children, no matter how she felt about anything they did. Regardless of the mechanical factors that may have developed in her jaw, it seemed clear that this was the real reason for this woman's TMJ problem. She would probably continue to experience it, no matter what treatment she received, until this aspect of her life changed. She was literally "biting back" angry words all of the time, until the muscles of her jaw had become locked into this habit.

All myofascial pain syndromes share certain basic similarities, and in my own practice, I have had good results in treating these conditions with acupuncture. Massage can also be effective, as can certain physical exercises or breathing techniques. All of these involve the release of muscle tension through direct physical stimulation of the body. Sometimes, muscular tension release will be accompanied by emotional release as well. Stimulation of critical points with acupuncture needles or deep massage may bring up thoughts, images, or emotions that are associated with the existing tension.

This can be physically and emotionally painful, but also highly therapeutic. One woman who had extremely tight muscles began to cry during her first acupuncture treatment. She told me later that when she returned home, she continued to cry uncontrollably for hours. Afterward she felt an enormous sense of release. On her next visit she seemed much more relaxed, and her muscles were obviously softer to the touch. She received several more treatments, during which her whole condition seemed to be transformed, both physically and emotionally.

Another woman treated with acupuncture for TMJ syndrome had an interesting response. Following her treatment, she found herself saying things to people that she would normally have held back. Her jaw felt a lot better, but she had to be careful to watch what she was saying for fear of speaking too freely. The physical release of tension in the muscles accompanied the release of a certain blockage in her behavior. Now she had to learn to control her words without locking them in with spasm of her jaw muscles.

Letting Go of Pain

While physical techniques such as acupuncture or massage can be very effective for relief of myofascial pain, other treatment may also be needed. Deborah and Kathy were women in their late twenties who consulted me at almost the same time with remarkably similar stories. Both had been involved in nearly identical automobile accidents several months previously. Each of them had been hit from behind and experienced typical "whiplash" injury to the neck, for which they received the usual treatment of rest, pain pills, muscle relaxants, and physical therapy.

X-rays showed nothing more than continued muscle spasm, but they both continued to hurt. Though they had shown some improvement, after several months these women were still taking pain medication every day and were unable to resume a normal life. They were beginning to wonder when they would ever get over their injuries, and had come to me to see if there were possibilities for treatment beyond conventional medical care.

I put them both on essentially the same program. This consisted of regular sessions of acupuncture and massage, along with exercises to loosen the neck muscles and restore flexibility. They were also taught some relaxation techniques to practice at home. Deborah did very well and each week felt a definite improvement. After two months her symptoms were nearly gone. She was enormously relieved to be free of pain, and told us she wished she had come sooner, rather than struggling with her problem for months. It was a very satisfying outcome for everyone involved in her care.

Kathy's response to the very same course of treatment was much less satisfying. She enjoyed her visits to the office, and after each treatment she would leave feeling more comfortable than when she arrived. But each time she returned, she complained that the pain was again as bad as before. Sometimes she would seem to make real progress for a while, but then there would be a setback and all at once she would be worse again. I continued to see Kathy for quite some time, but eventually it became apparent that she was not going to get better with what we were doing.

Deborah, the first patient, was able to get better once she received effective treatment. There was no reason for her to continue to have pain. But Kathy's situation was different. Although her problem had begun in the same way, it had eventually taken on another dimension and become more complicated. The pain in her neck was no longer merely the physical result of a whiplash injury. It had also become the focus of all the emotional pain in her life, of which there was a great deal. Even before the accident, Kathy had felt dissatisfied with her life, and every unhappy event now triggered increased pain and spasm in her neck.

Unfortunately this was difficult for her to recognize, and even more difficult for her to acknowledge to others. She continued to insist that her neck pain was a purely physical problem caused by the auto accident, and had nothing to do with anything else in her life.

As time went by, Kathy's symptoms also served an additional purpose. Her chronic pain became a source of attention and sympathy from other people. While it was not acceptable for her to complain that her life was un-happy, she felt free to talk to people about how much her neck hurt and thus receive their sympathy. Her medical problem also provided a legitimate reason to take time off

from her job, which she disliked. If she did not want to go
to work, the easiest way to accomplish this was to have her
neck pain flare up, although she may not have con-
sciously admitted this to herself.

Kathy was also pursuing a lawsuit against the other
driver in the accident for a large settlement. Lawsuits
often prove to be a real obstacle to the patient's full recovery. On some level, she feels that she must continue to
have pain until the lawsuit is settled, a process that can
frequently take years to complete.

For Kathy, the lawsuit also provided a way to blame
someone else for her problems. Instead of examining how
she may have created unhappiness in her life, she could
blame it all on her condition and those involved in it: the
driver who caused the accident, the doctors who could not
seem to cure her, the insurance companies that were so
slow to respond, the lawyers who would not give her a
direct answer—in short, she could blame everyone but
herself.

There was no real difference in the physical injuries
experienced by Deborah and Kathy. But Deborah had no
reason not to get well, while the reasons for Kathy to hold
onto her pain eventually outweighed the reasons to give it
up. The pain had become the focus of her life. And as long
as this was true, there was no way that I, or any other
doctor, would be able to help her.

Pain and tension in the muscular system can be the
expression of both physical and emotional problems in
the life of the patient. In order for these symptoms to be
resolved, it may be necessary to address them on different
levels. For some people, therapies that work directly on
the physical body, such as acupuncture, therapeutic massage, or exercise, may give excellent results; at times,
these may be all that is needed for the patient to get well.
For others, it may also be necessary to recognize, and to
explore in more depth, the emotional causes that can
underlie physical symptoms.

Human beings are complex; the condition of a person's physical body and his or her emotional state are frequently intertwined. Therefore, it is up to the doctor to provide treatment for all the different aspects of a medical problem. And it is up to the patient to provide a willingness to let go of the symptoms and allow himself to get well.

6

Avoiding the Hazards
of Modern Medicine

Staying Out of the Hospital

As a medical student, I occasionally encountered patients
who were very wary of doctors. Usually they were older
people who had never had much to do with doctors, but
had at last been driven to seek medical care for some
problem they could not manage. I remember one elderly
man who was told he would need to be admitted to the
hospital. He was very reluctant to agree and offered many
reasons why it would be difficult for him to leave his
home. As we continued to insist that he be admitted so
that we could help him, it eventually became clear that he
was terrified to enter the hospital.

He had never been in a hospital, and he believed it was
a place in which people died. We all assured him that he
had the wrong idea entirely, and as we discussed it later,
our attitude toward this nice old man was one of affection-
ate amusement. How foolish and old-fashioned it was for
someone nowadays to be afraid of going into the hospital.
After all, hospitals were places where people went to get
better.

Now, as I recall this incident from a more mature
perspective, I can see that this man was not as foolish as

we thought. Modern medicine has powerful techniques to cure, but these techniques can also do harm if something goes awry. And in the increasingly complex world of medical technology it is all too easy for something to go wrong. Although hospitals *are* places where people can get better, they can also be dangerous. Unforeseen and sometimes serious things happen to people in hospitals that would not happen at home, and they are places that are best avoided unless absolutely essential.

A Medical Casualty

I served my internship in a hospital that possessed a feature not often found today. This was a tuberculosis ward. Even at the time it was something of a throwback to the past. Tucked away on the top floor, and quite separate from most other activities in the building, it was devoted solely to the care of patients with active tuberculosis who were too contagious to leave the hospital and mingle in society. Almost all were men, most of them poor, with a significant number of the homeless or derelict among them.

There was a curious ambiguity about the status of these patients. On the one hand, they were in the hospital because they had a serious illness that required long-term treatment. Yet they were also there because they represented a threat to the public health, so that a certain element of coercion was entailed in keeping them confined until the doctors decided they were no longer sufficiently contagious to endanger others.

Because tuberculosis is slow to resolve, most of the people admitted to this ward remained for a long time. While the progress of other patients was measured in days, theirs was more often measured in weeks or even months. However, none of them were acutely ill, so the doctors assigned to the ward kept regular nine-to-five hours. At all other times, the intern on duty for the regular medical wards was also responsible for the tuberculosis patients, although he was rarely needed. Thus, while on call one weekend at the hospital, I was surprised to hear myself paged for the tuberculosis ward. When I arrived, the nurse asked me to look at a patient who had just been admitted that day and was complaining of pain in his hand.

He was an older, disheveled-looking man who appeared agitated and confused, and apparently spoke no English. He was speaking rapidly in Portuguese, and gesturing repeatedly with his other hand at the hand that bothered him. I could not understand what he was saying, but examined his hand carefully. It appeared entirely normal. I saw no swelling or bruising, and it did not seem to hurt when I pushed on it. Finally, I decided there could be nothing seriously wrong with his hand. Whatever it was could certainly wait for his regular doctor the next morning, and I returned to more pressing problems elsewhere in the hospital.

The next evening I was again surprised to hear a page from the tuberculosis ward. It was for the same patient. That morning, the doctors on the ward had decided to order an X-ray of his hand. This had revealed a hairline fracture that was too slight to require treatment, and in fact no longer seemed to be bothering him much. Now he was complaining about pain in his hip. Once again, communication was difficult, but I learned from the nurses that he had apparently fallen while waiting to have his hand X-rayed. I again examined him and found nothing obviously wrong, and decided that this problem too could wait for the morning.

This time when he was sent for X-rays, they revealed a more serious problem. He had a fractured hip, presumably sustained when he had fallen the day before. Now he was temporarily transferred from the tuberculosis ward to the surgery department, and a repair of his hip was scheduled. The surgery itself went smoothly, but as he was coming out of general anaesthesia, he suffered a cardiac arrest.

After a prolonged effort, he was finally resuscitated in the operating room. However, he did not awaken from the anaesthesia and remained in a coma. There was nothing more the surgeons could do so he was again transferred, this time to the general medical ward. At this point he officially became my patient. We did our best for him, but despite our efforts his condition went downhill rapidly and he died several days later without ever awakening.

I felt there was a kind of irony that he had come to die under my care. Through a curious chain of circumstances, I had been involved in each step leading from his admission to the hospital to his death from a totally unrelated cause only a week later. It was likely that nobody else had seen his story unfold so clearly, and I could not help but wonder about what I had seen. Although each of the medical decisions made in his case was apparently correct in itself, together they had somehow led to his death. Why did this happen?

Certainly nobody could have known he would fall in the X-ray department or have a cardiac arrest in surgery. Nevertheless, these events had happened, and they are typical of things that *do* seem to happen to people in hospitals. If he had not been in the hospital, or if his doctors had not X-rayed his hand, none of the subsequent events would have taken place and he would still have been alive. With the best of intentions, his medical care had killed him. It was a case of what we now refer to as *iatrogenic* disease—a term that is coming into increasing use to describe the growing problem of disease produced solely as a consequence of medical care.

This story is particularly striking in its progression from a trivial injury to cardiac arrest and death. But it is not a unique story. Although not always so dramatic, it is not that unusual for medical intervention to lead to new problems that are sometimes more serious than the original ones. There are definitely hazards associated with medical care that go along with its benefits. Sometimes they take the form of unexpected, almost random events, as in this case. At other times, they are more predictable.

Treatment Can Be More Dangerous Than the Disease

Mrs. Johnson was a woman in her late fifties with rheumatoid arthritis. For many years she had been treated with Prednisone—a steroid drug related to cortisone. Although such drugs often relieve the symptoms of arthritis, they can also have serious side effects. One of the most well known side effects of prolonged steroid therapy is osteoporosis, a generalized loss of calcium that leads to thinning and weakening of the bones. Osteoporosis causes bones to break more easily, and this is what had happened to Mrs. Johnson. After years of steroid therapy, several of the vertebrae in her spine had literally collapsed. The result was severe, unremitting pain in her back, far worse than any pain she ever experienced with arthritis, which is what the steroids had been prescribed to treat.

There was extensive and irreversible structural damage to her spine, and there was little I could offer in the way of real help with her pain. I felt saddened by her situation and by the thought that after years of medical care, involving great time and expense, she would probably be better off now if she had never seen a doctor over the past twenty years.

Mrs. Fields, another patient with a similarly unfortunate story, was a woman in her sixties with chronic pain in her leg. Her problems had begun several years previously, when she consulted her doctor about occasional episodes of dizziness. He thought they might be caused by partial obstruction of the arteries in her neck, and to investigate this further an arteriogram was performed. This is a procedure in which dye is injected into the blood vessels and a series of X-rays is then taken.

It is an excellent technique for evaluating the condition of the arteries, but it is not entirely without risk. A small percentage of people who have arteriograms will experience complications, and unfortunately Mrs. Fields was one of these. Following injection of the dye into her arteries, she suffered a stroke that left one side of her body partially paralyzed.

This was a tremendous blow, but she had a lot of spirit, and despite the stroke, she was soon up and around again, walking with the help of a cane. However, she may have tried to be up too soon, because not long afterward, she fell while walking with her cane and fractured her hip. Now she required surgery to repair her hip, and although it seemed to heal well, she was left with chronic pain in her hip and leg and could no longer walk, even with a cane.

When I saw her several years after all of this had happened, her condition was not good. She had become an invalid, confined to her bed most of the time. She was chronically depressed and dependent upon pain pills. Clearly, she would have been much better off simply living with an occasional dizzy spell than becoming involved in this course of events.

Then there was the young man who complained to his doctor of pain in some of his joints. No diagnosis was clearly made, but he was routinely prescribed an anti-inflammatory drug commonly used to treat arthritis. He soon began to experience symptoms of intestinal irritation from this drug. As he continued to take the medication, this condition quickly progressed to a bleeding ulcer. He was hospitalized on an emergency basis with a major hemorrhage, and, at the age of twenty-five, had part of his stomach surgically removed.

Whether he ever actually had arthritis was not clear, but he certainly did have a very real problem as a result of the treatment. He survived and eventually made a full recovery, but he was left with an abiding skepticism about using drugs and the wisdom of the doctors who prescribe them.

A somewhat different story involved a man in his forties who suffered from low back pain. His doctors were unable to find anything obviously wrong with his back, but he continued to complain that it hurt. It seemed that something further must be done, and it was decided to perform a myelogram, an X-ray procedure that involves injection of dye into the spinal canal. The X-rays showed no abnormality, but the patient had an inflammatory reaction to the dye. As a result, he developed a condition called "adhesive arachnoiditis," in which fibrous adhesions form along the lining of the spinal cord and nerve roots.

This condition now caused constant, severe pain, far worse than his original back pain. It was also extremely difficult to treat. A more thoughtful evaluation at the onset of his pain might have revealed some factors in his life that were contributing to his persistent back pain. But now he had irreversible damage to his spinal canal, and it was too late for such an evaluation. In fact, it was not clear what to do for him now, and he was left to make the rounds of the pain clinics, in search of something that could help.

These stories are all anecdotes. They are a few examples of individual people who have experienced unfortunate results from drugs or conventional medical care. They are not statistics, and do not reflect how often this sort of thing happens. But I think they convey better than any statistics the human dimensions of what can occur when medical care does not go as planned. And I suspect that these problems happen more often than we would like to believe. I regret to say that I could easily relate a good many other similar stories.

Why does iatrogenic illness occur so frequently? To some extent, it is an unavoidable consequence of today's medical system. We have powerful drugs and highy effective procedures for accomplishing certain ends. However, the very power of these techniques is intrinsically dangerous. The serious side effects are the other side of the benefits they make available.

Whenever we turn to the positive benefits of modern medicine, we must be prepared to expect at least some risks as well. However, these risks do not have to be as prevalent as they seem to have become. We need an approach to medicine that will still make available the benefits of medical technology, while minimizing the risk to the patient.

The Dangers of Medication

Many problems inherent in medical care stem from the idea that the doctor must *do* something for the patient. This is not entirely the doctor's fault. Often the patient may not feel satisfied that anything has been accomplished unless he leaves the doctor's office with some concrete "treatment." Typically, this takes the form of a prescription for medication.

Sometimes this may be appropriate. A patient with pneumonia, for example, may get over the illness on his own, but he will do so much faster and more comfortably with a prescription for an antibiotic. Similarly, someone who has just strained his back and is experiencing severe muscle spasm will feel better with rest. But if he has intense pain, a couple of pain pills may make him much more comfortable while he is resting.

I see nothing wrong with prescribing drugs in these situations. In both cases, the drug is used to treat an acute problem and is discontinued as soon as the patient is better. The drug is used solely to speed the healing proc-

ess or make the patient more comfortable, and it is unlikely to create serious side effects.

However, many drugs are prescribed for a prolonged
period of time, which creates quite a different situation. If
the patient with back spasm continues to take pain pills,
and the days stretch into weeks or even months, these
drugs are no longer helping him to get well. More likely
they are suppressing a symptom that calls for some response. And the longer they are taken, the more they are
liable to lead to side effects.

Drugs such as pain pills or tranquilizers pose the additional problem of dependence. As the medication is continued, the body develops a tolerance for its effects, so that
increasingly high doses become necessary to produce the
same result. And as tolerance increases, the patient also
develops a dependence upon continued use of the drug. If
he attempts to stop, he must now contend with the problem of withdrawal.

Other drugs, while not addicting in the same sense,
can also create dependence. By continually suppressing
the symptoms of illness, they prevent the patient from
ever making the response that is needed to resolve the
illness. The treatment itself thus helps to create a self-
perpetuating condition that continues to call for more
treatment.

A good example of this effect can be seen among
patients with asthma. These people experience bronchospasm, a constriction of the breathing passages of the
lungs. In order to reverse this, they are usually treated
with drugs that stimulate the breathing passages to open.
While these drugs do work, they must be taken continuously to control bronchospasm. But as they reverse the
symptoms, they also remove the opportunity for the
body's own mechanisms of regulation to respond to these
symptoms and restore a more normal state. The symptoms then persist, and before long, the patient is stuck on
a treadmill of indefinite drug therapy that may actually
help to perpetuate the illness.

I was particularly impressed by one young woman who was taking a remarkable number of asthma medications. She took four kinds of bronchodilators several times a day in pill form, as well as three different inhalers, and for the past several months had also been receiving Prednisone, a cortisone-like drug that is often the final step in attempting to control asthma. All these medications had been prescribed by her doctor, who had continued to add one new drug after another. Despite all the medication, she was still having difficulty breathing.

But how could she ever expect to get well again with so many different drugs circulating in her body? Her body could not return to normal, or even recognize any longer what "normal" would be, with so many drugs exerting their various influences. Although she was taking more drugs than most people with asthma, it is not unusual for other patients to be prescribed a similar collection of medications.

Clearly drugs are necessary at times. When a patient is gasping for breath, both he and his doctor need some way to intervene that will be immediately effective. But while doctors will give out prescriptions freely, they may not give enough thought to how their patients are going to get off medication once they have begun—or to the possible side effects of long-term multiple drug therapy.

Medical Decisions

In addition to prescribing drugs, another thing doctors regularly *do* for their patients is order tests. Laboratory tests are a vital part of medicine, but sometimes too many can be ordered and they create problems of their own. Tests may turn up unexpected abnormalities, which must then be pursued further, and soon the patient has become ensnared in the hazards of modern health care.

Mr. Barnwell was a college professor in his late thirties who had always been in good health and visited the doctor conscientiously every year for an annual checkup. Following one of these, he was surprised to learn that his routine lab work had shown some abnormalities. Although he felt completely well, several blood tests of liver function were mildly elevated and he was told by his doctor to return and have them repeated in a month.

A month later the tests were still abnormal, and this time his doctor recommended a liver biopsy. This involves inserting a large needle through the wall of the abdomen into the liver, and then withdrawing a sample of tissue to be examined. A biopsy is the most direct way of diagnosing any liver problem, but it is also an uncomfortable procedure that is not entirely without risk. Although it is reasonably safe when done by an experienced physician, occasionally a patient will experience internal bleeding or some other complication.

Mr. Barnwell agonized over his doctor's advice for a while. He understood what a liver biopsy was, and really did not want to have one, especially as he felt completely well. However, he did not want to go against his doctor's advice, and he was afraid of leaving some serious problem undiagnosed. Eventually he came to me for another opinion. Did I think he needed a liver biopsy or not?

I reviewed his lab tests, and advised him to simply wait. If anything really was wrong with him, it would soon become more apparent. On the other hand, people sometimes have unexplained changes in liver tests that are probably the result of some illness too mild to be noticed. If this was the case for Mr. Barnwell, there was certainly no point in putting him through a liver biopsy. We could just check his lab tests periodically and make sure they returned to normal. If not, there was time to think about a biopsy later.

Mr. Barnwell received my opinion with great relief. Over the next five months, we watched his liver function tests return completely to normal, while he continued to feel well. There was no need for a liver biopsy, and if he had not happened to have some routine blood tests, neither he nor anyone else would ever have known anything was wrong. He was happy with the outcome, and I was glad to have saved him an unnecessary stay in the hospital.

Medical practice often involves making similar judgments. When a patient is seriously ill, it is clear that something must be done, and the doctor must be prepared to act decisively. But many situations require a more considered judgment. There is no clear right or wrong way to proceed. The benefits must be balanced against the risks to arrive at the best course of action. Should the doctor treat the patient now or wait a couple of days to see how he does? Should the patient be admitted to the hospital, or can he be allowed to remain at home? Should a battery of lab tests be ordered at once, or can the patient be given only a few basic ones at first?

These kinds of questions arise repeatedly in medical practice. It would not really have been *wrong* to perform a liver biopsy on Mr. Barnwell. He had an unexplained abnormality, and a biopsy is the most direct way to arrive at a diagnosis. But while it was not wrong, the hazards of a liver biopsy far outweighed the benefits in this situation. It seemed better for Mr. Barnwell to simply wait and see what happened.

It is remarkable how often this can be the best course of action. Time is a wonderful healer, and the physician need not always feel compelled to jump in and *do* something immediately. Repeatedly, I find myself saying to patients, "I could treat you now, but let's wait a couple of days and we may not need to do anything," or "I think your lab tests will be normal, so let's wait a little before we order any," or other words to this effect. Often the problem does indeed take care of itself without any intervention from the doctor.

The best way I know of deciding what to do for a patient is to consider what I would do in his place. What if I had the same symptom myself—or if it was my father or my wife or my child sitting across the desk from me with the problem? I know that if I had been in Mr. Barnwell's position, I would not have wanted a liver biopsy. And I wonder if the physician who was so ready to perform one on Mr. Barnwell would have been as prepared to have one himself in the same circumstances.

Childbirth as a Medical Event

One of the reasons for the growing number of problems associated with medical care is that people today turn to doctors and hospitals far more often than they did in the past. Although in certain areas of life we are all prepared to accept the authority of physicians, somehow doctors have gradually extended their authority into areas that individuals once managed on their own. Thus, people have ceased to take personal responsibility for themselves and instead take on the role of "patient." Perhaps nowhere is this more apparent today than in the process of childbirth.

In most traditional cultures, the supervision of childbirth has, for obvious reasons, been the province of women. In some cultures, men not only do not supervise childbirth, but are excluded from all aspects of it. The time of labor is often a time for men to step aside as women take care of what is, biologically, the concern of women. It is only in modern technological societies that male physicians have taken over this traditionally female role, and I suspect that people in some traditional cultures might find the idea of a male doctor delivering babies rather bizarre.

The supervision of childbirth by physicians, and especially male physicians, has changed the quality of this experience for women today. In response to this change there has recently been a movement by women to regain their role in childbirth by recalling the profession of midwife. Although they were not long ago an accepted part of society, today the legal status of midwives is vague, and often they seem to face more hostility than cooperation from the established medical profession. Midwives have been prosecuted for practicing medicine without a license, and in at least one case, even charged with murder for attending at a childbirth in which the baby did not live.

Regardless of how one feels about midwives, it is an interesting statement about our times that someone could be prosecuted for practicing medicine without a license for attending at childbirth. This indicates how thoroughly we have accepted the idea that childbirth is a *medical* event. We take it as a matter of course that this aspect of life should be under the supervision of doctors, and that they may establish rules for how it takes place.

When I was an intern being trained in obstetrics, I was taught to approach childbirth as one would a surgical procedure. All patients routinely had their pelvic areas shaved and cleaned, and a great deal of attention was given to maintaining sterile technique during the delivery. Every patient entered the delivery room with an IV needle already in her arm, in case any unexpected problems should arise, and the doctor was carefully clothed in sterile gown, mask, and gloves before he even went into the room.

Prior to delivery, patients in labor were examined periodically to check on their progress. Anyone who was screaming a lot or complaining of much pain would get a shot of Demerol. Although Demerol or other narcotics will depress the life functions of the baby, several of these shots were sometimes given during the course of labor. As long as nobody seemed to get an unreasonably high dosage, there was no serious concern.

Given the atmosphere in the labor rooms, it is not surprising that narcotics were used so routinely. For both patients and staff alike, a couple of shots of Demerol seemed like a better alternative than hours of pain and hysterical screaming. The idea that the mother might learn to manage what she was feeling without the need for drugs was never seriously considered.

At the time of delivery, additional drugs were usually administered, often as injections of anaesthetic around the cervix. When the baby was born, it would be slapped a bit to induce a cry; I would congratulate the mother, tell her if it was a boy or girl, and hold the baby up for her to see. A nurse would then promptly whisk it away to the nursery, and although the baby had just come out of the mother's body, she was not permitted to touch it, even for a moment, in deference to some vaguely defined concern with infection.

I do not think anyone really questioned this extraordinary prohibition against a mother touching her newborn child. It was simply accepted as one of the rules to be followed. This practice clearly prevented the mother from putting the child on her breast to nurse, but it was generally assumed that women did not want to breastfeed their babies anyway. Unless a specific request to breastfeed was made, mothers were routinely given a hormone injection immediately after delivery to dry up their breasts.

Thus, women presented themselves at the hospital at the onset of labor as passive participants in the process of birth, and there was no attempt by the hospital staff to change this attitude. It was assumed by all concerned that it was the doctor, and not the mother, who would assume responsibility for whatever happened in the hospital. Since that time, things have changed for the better. A movement toward greater awareness of the quality of childbirth has prompted many doctors and hospitals to modify their procedures.

However, hospital births are still approached on primarily medical grounds. While this approach has the advantage of minimizing certain risks, it has also diminished the quality of the experience. The drugged woman in the hospital delivery room is no longer an individual going through an intense and meaningful experience in her life, but a patient with a medical condition who is under the care of a doctor.

Unforeseen Hazards of Medical Intervention

A hospital childbirth assisted by modern technology is designed to prevent as many medical problems as possible. However, the use of medical technology where it may not be necessary can lead indirectly to new problems. A good example is the use of the fetal monitor. As the name implies, this is a device that monitors the condition of the baby in the uterus by recording its heart rate. By indicating a change in heart rate, the fetal monitor has the advantage of allowing the doctor to quickly recognize possible fetal distress. He can then intervene and deliver the baby by Caesarian section, which, if done promptly, can prevent damage to the baby. But due to a curious combination of circumstances, use of the fetal monitor can also lead to its own complications.

The doctor can never be faulted for performing a Caesarian section if there is any question of a problem. However, he can very definitely be blamed, both medically and legally, for *not* doing this, if there is any subsequent damage to the baby.

In recent years, this issue has arisen in major malpractice judgments against doctors attending at births. Thus, powerful pressures influence the doctor to deliver the baby surgically at the first sign of any trouble. Because any abnormality on the monitor may be interpreted in retrospect as evidence of a problem, its use intensifies the pressure on the doctor to act immediately. As a result, widespread use of the fetal monitor may be one of the factors contributing to the enormous increase in Caesarian sections being performed.

At some hospitals today, at least one in three babies is born by Caesarian section, and the rate continues to climb. This is a relatively new phenomenon. Until quite recently, Caesarian section was not a common procedure. Most women managed to have their babies safely without it, as women still do throughout much of the rest of the world. For most of this century, the rate of Caesarian section in this country remained fairly constant at approximately two to four percent of all births. This rate persisted in most hospitals until as recently as thirty years ago. Thus, the magnitude of increase for Caesarian sections over the last thirty years has been monumental.

The reasons for this increase are complex. Undoubtedly some of the women now having Caesarian sections could eventually have had a normal delivery, had there been no intervention. This may be particularly true when the doctor elects to intervene too quickly in response to transient changes in heart rate on the monitor. In this way, a device designed to make childbirth safer may paradoxically increase the number of mothers and babies being subjected to surgery. For at least some of these women, it might have proved safer to have their baby unassisted by all the technological advantages of the hospital.

Do the dangers prevented by fetal monitors justify the dangers of unnecessary intervention that result from their routine use? I do not have the answer to this question, but it is the sort of question that must be seriously considered before indiscriminately embracing any technological innovation in medical care, especially when it involves a normal biological activity such as childbirth. The advantages of medical intervention are often obvious and dramatic, but the disadvantages that go along with them may be easy to overlook.

Clearly there are situations in which intervention with the full range of medical technology is not only desirable, but necessary to safeguard the life of both mother and baby. However, an approach to childbirth focused only on getting the baby out alive, while ignoring the emotional and spiritual qualities of the experience, reduces the scope of our lives as human beings. We need a greater balance in our medical system, so that hospitals and medical technology can be readily available when needed, but do not intrude on a natural, biological function.

Taking Responsibility for Health

Although it is particularly obvious in the case of childbirth, in many other areas of our lives we have given up our capacity to make decisions about our health and medical care. Instead we have handed over this authority to doctors. As we have seen, this abandonment of personal responsibility can lead to unfortunate results.

Doctors possess information and skills unavailable to their patients, but this does not necessarily ensure that their decisions will always be best for another individual. Thus, there may be times when it is up to the patient to protect himself against the excesses of modern medical care. This means giving serious consideration to what the doctor advises, but remaining open to questioning this advice and not necessarily accepting all his conclusions as correct.

Often no simple, right answer to a medical problem is available; the patient may be offered only judgments. One doctor's judgment may not be the same as another's, and neither may concur with what the patient feels is best for himself. Doctors provide essential information for an informed decision, but ultimately this decision is up to the individual.

If a doctor says you should have this test done, or take that drug, or have this operation, he is offering his best judgment. However, your idea of the risks and benefits involved may be different from his. It is your health and life, and you must choose a course that will leave you feeling better as a result of medical care, rather than with worse problems than when you began.

Modern hospitals and medical technology have become an integral part of our lives. They have great power to help us, but they can also do us harm. We would certainly not want to do without them, yet we should approach them with respect, and become involved with them only when it becomes absolutely necessary.

PART TWO

EXPLORING ALTERNATIVES IN MEDICINE

7

Hypnosis, Suggestion, and the Process of Healing

Life and Death Beliefs

The first time I heard a patient told he was going to die I was in my third year of medical school. Until then my education had consisted of sitting in a classroom listening to lectures about medicine, and I was now beginning the major transition of actually applying some of what I had learned to real patients. The general medical ward to which I was assigned, at the nearby Veterans Hospital, averaged about thirty patients who presented a great variety of medical problems.

Mr. Baxter, a recent admission to the ward, was a quiet, slender man in his early fifties who worked as a salesman. Mr. Baxter had a cough. He also complained of feeling tired all the time and had experienced an unexplained loss of weight over the past couple of months. He had smoked two packs of cigarettes a day for better than thirty years, so we all had a bad feeling about his cough. When he was admitted, he underwent the usual routine of examinations, laboratory tests, and X-rays, and within a few days we had a diagnosis.

As expected, Mr. Baxter had lung cancer. It had already spread from his lungs to other parts of his body, and he was beyond the point where surgery could help. Chemotherapy and radiotherapy were also ruled out as options for treatment. We felt these would only subject him to very unpleasant side-effects without significantly altering his illness. There was nothing we could do but break the news and send him home.

When we made the rounds of our patients the next morning, I felt a nervous anticipation as we reached Mr. Baxter's room. Our entire group—medical resident, two interns, and two medical students—all dressed in long white coats with stethoscopes in our pockets, entered the room and gathered around his bed as we did every morning. As senior member of the team, our resident took charge of the situation. He was a serious, heavyset young man, who seemed to think of nothing but medicine; in fact, I was somewhat in awe of his encyclopedic knowledge of the subject. He spoke quietly for a few moments, explaining to Mr. Baxter what we had found. He told him we proposed to discharge him from the hospital the following day.

Mr. Baxter heard him through without interruption, and when he was finished asked how long he could expect to live. He was told that he had about four months. After hearing this, he calmly thanked us for all we had done. Throughout the conversation, he had remained serious but composed.

As we filed out of the room again, I marveled at the scene I had just witnessed. It had seemed more like something seen in a movie or television program than anything in my own experience. As a young medical student, I was impressed by how the resident had handled himself in this difficult situation, and I wondered if I would ever be able to do as well myself. I was also impressed by how well the patient had behaved in receiving such devastating information.

Yet as I look back on this scene now, I see another dimension to what took place that I was entirely unaware of at that time. I realize that Mr. Baxter was not merely receiving objective information from his doctor. He was also receiving the enormously powerful suggestion that he was going to die in four months. At this critical moment, when he was intensely receptive to everything being said, this suggestion was deeply implanted in him. I do not know what happened to him after he left the hospital, but I would be surprised if he lived more than four months—not only because he had widespread cancer, but also because he had accepted death in four months as the inescapable outcome of his illness.

As a figure of supreme authority, the doctor is in a position to provide suggestions of great power with his every word. If he says you will die in four months, and you accept this, your body may make the necessary physiological adjustments so that this is indeed what happens. The doctor's words then become a self-fulfilling prophecy.

There are stories of people in primitive societies who have died with no demonstrable cause other than the curse of a witch doctor. Their belief in the power of the witch doctor was apparently so strong that their physical bodies were actually affected to the point that death occurred. Although we may not appreciate comparison with a witch doctor, the dynamics of the situation are fundamentally no different when a modern physician tells a patient he is going to die.

Like most people, Mr. Baxter was not prepared to challenge what he was told by his doctor. It would have taken someone of unusual personal strength to do so in these circumstances. Anyone who has been a patient in a hospital will appreciate that it is an experience structured to eliminate one's capacity for independent decision.

The hospital patient is routinely told by others when to sleep or wake up, what to eat, and what he must do all day. His regular clothes are taken away, and he is placed in a room where his normal privacy is continually invaded. He is typically subjected to tests and procedures that are uncomfortable, mysterious, and often intimidating. He is poked with needles and prodded with tubes, but no matter what is done to him, he must continue to do as he is told for it has all been ordered by the doctor. He repeatedly finds himself in situations that would be unacceptable in almost any other setting.

At last, the critical moment arrives when he is to learn what the doctors have determined. He is lying in bed, dressed only in hospital pajamas, while they stand over him in a circle. They are fully dressed in the medical uniforms that symbolize special status and knowledge. When they deliver their judgment, it carries the full weight of their profession.

How could anyone expect the patient to seriously question what he is told? It would be difficult to imagine circumstances more conducive to helplessness. Yet what is remarkable in this scene, and countless others like it, is that everyone seems totally unaware there is even an element of suggestion involved. They are under the illusion that what is happening is simply an objective transmission of information. With the best of intentions, the doctor believes he is only telling the patient how long a man with metastatic lung cancer of a certain stage can normally expect to live.

But obviously there is more taking place. The patient is also receiving a particular set of beliefs about the condition of his body. How much is the outcome of his illness determined by his physical condition, and how much by what he *believes* about this condition? What if Mr. Baxter had been told he could expect to live another six months rather than four? Would he have been more likely to live a little longer? Or what if he had been told that he would live for several years, or even that he was not going to die from his cancer at all? How would these different expectations have altered the physical process taking place in his body?

Certainly this cannot be carried too far. We could not responsibly have told Mr. Baxter that everything was going to be fine, no matter how positive a suggestion this would be. Yet there have undoubtedly been people with the same disease who have lived longer than four months. Probably some may have lived for years, and perhaps even a rare few recovered from their disease and apparently got well again. We refer to such unexpected recoveries as "spontaneous remissions." Although their cause remains a mystery, spontaneous remissions seem to occur most often among people who believe they can get well.

The same illness will not follow an identical course in every patient. Thus, the doctor's prediction of how long Mr. Baxter would live was no more than a well-informed guess. Yet it was presented in such a way as to preclude the possibility of a more successful outcome. It would not have been fair to give Mr. Baxter a falsely optimistic picture, but it was also unfair to convey a sense of total hopelessness to him. Doctors can only provide statistical probabilities based on past experience. No doctor, however well informed, can tell a patient with complete certainty that there is no chance for him to get well.

At all levels of medical care, a quality of communication is needed that gives the patient realistic information, yet still leaves open at least some possibility of hope. If his belief can help him die in four months, then a more positive belief may also help him *not* die in this time. Unfortunately, the power of belief to alter the state of the physical body is often ignored in medical practice.

Positive Versus Negative Suggestions

Doctors not only miss the opportunity to instill positive beliefs in their patients, they may also make negative suggestions without even realizing they are doing so. This need not be as dramatic as telling a patient he is going to die soon. It can occur with anything a doctor tells a patient about his condition.

I have seen many patients with chronic pain problems that are frustrating for a physician to treat. Sometimes the doctor's frustration at his inability to help may be communicated to the patients in the form of negative suggestions. They may be told "You will have this pain for the rest of your life," or "There is nothing more that can be done for you," or other words to this effect. These words cause the patient to believe that he can never get better, and this, in turn, becomes an enormously difficult obstacle to overcome in future treatment.

Of course, what the doctor really means is "There is nothing more that *I* can do for you." This is a crucial distinction, because it implies that even though one doctor was unable to help, there is still the possibility that someone else may be successful. I often find it essential to convince patients in this situation that this is what is actually being said, and that it remains possible for them to be helped in some way.

I have seen patients conditioned by their doctors to believe in limits to their ability to get well that do not really exist. Mr. James was a man in his early sixties with chronic neck and shoulder pain. I had been treating him with acupuncture with some success. His X-rays were only mildly abnormal and I felt it was possible for him to get over his pain completely. However, he had been told by another doctor some years earlier that the vertebrae in his neck were "crushed" and he would always be in pain as a result. This image had become firmly lodged in his mind. Repeatedly, he would tell me how much better he was feeling, and then go on to assure me ". . . of course, I can never expect to get rid of all this pain because my vertebrae are 'crushed.' "

My suggestion that his X-rays did not look all that bad was not able to budge his firmly held image of the condition of his neck. His other physician had actually been quite skillful at suggestion, and in a brief conversation had managed to give Mr. James a compelling image that remained with him for years. Unfortunately, the nature of this suggestion had been quite destructive. Had this physician been more aware of the effect of his words, he could easily have chosen to convey a more positive image to his patient.

Negative suggestions may be more profound than simply a thoughtless choice of words. Sometimes I am appalled at the things people are told by their doctors. Paula was an overweight young woman who had suffered from low back pain for several years. Two years before I saw her, she had been hospitalized for evaluation. Although nothing specific had been found, she was told "Your back will continue to get worse and in a couple of years you will need an operation." What a terrible prediction to make. The problem with her back was now compounded by her anxiety about this suggestion.

Fortunately, Paula had never totally accepted the idea that she was bound to get worse. I assured her that I could see no basis for such a dire prediction, and that it seemed possible she could resolve her problem. She began a program that entailed a change in diet and exercise, and as she lost weight, she soon began to notice an improvement. Even more importantly, she was immensely relieved by a more optimistic prediction and was able to approach the whole situation with a changed attitude.

Another young woman who had undergone surgery for low back pain was told by the surgeon that she ". . . had the spine of an eighty-year-old woman," and would undoubtedly be back again for more surgery. This is an awful image to place in someone's mind about the condition of her body, and it was not even true. X-rays of her back did show more degeneration than expected for someone her age, but the surgeon's description was a great exaggeration.

Although she had tried to discount this evaluation, the image had stayed with her. She lived with the idea that her spine was severely and permanently damaged, and could easily be injured again at any time. Not surprisingly, she had a great deal of fear about the future, and was confused about what activities were safe for her. With a careless comment, her doctor had created a whole set of problems for her. As in the previous case, the most useful thing I could do was to reassure her and provide a more realistic, positive belief about the condition of her back and her future health.

These are not isolated instances, but a few particularly vivid examples of stories recounted by patients. Yet surely doctors do not intend to communicate with their patients in this destructive fashion. When this occurs, one can only assume they are unaware of the implications of their words. A fundamental precept of medical practice is that a doctor should *do no harm* in his treatment. It is necessary to remember that this applies as well to the use of words as to physical action.

Suggestion and Healing

The physician who *is* aware of his powers of suggestion can not only avoid suggesting negative outcomes to his patients, he can also use these powers to encourage positive results. When suggestion is used formally for this purpose, we call it hypnosis, but a great deal of more informal suggestion also takes place in medical practice. Elements of suggestion occur in every form of medical therapy, and although they may not call it by this name, or even be aware of what they are doing, physicians and other therapists often achieve their results by influencing the belief of their patients.

I have met therapists of all kinds who achieve successful outcomes with a wide variety of treatments. There are those who practice massage or manipulation, while others treat their patients with special diets or nutritional supplements. Some concentrate on different types of psychotherapy, or teach meditation or relaxation techniques. Others try to heal through movement, exercise, music, or herbs. There are psychic healers and faith healers, and those who attempt to manipulate the energy fields of the body. Many of these therapies offer intriguing possibilities that are neglected by conventional medicine; others are so implausible that even with the most open mind, I cannot accept that they have any objective effect.

Nevertheless, it is interesting that nearly all practitioners of alternative medicine, even the most bizarre, describe legitimate cases of people whom they have helped to resolve some illness. Perhaps part of the explanation is that there are more ways to influence the condition of the human organism than we may imagine. Beyond this, however, the success of so many different treatments has a common basis in the therapist's belief in his or her own ability. Any therapist who can effectively transmit this belief to the patient has taken a major step toward successfully healing that patient, regardless of the specific treatment used. The actual treatment itself may even be secondary to the patient's faith in its value.

It is easy to accept the importance of suggestion as a factor in unconventional forms of treatment. For example, skeptical observers have asked whether my whole practice of acupuncture is really nothing more than an elaborate form of suggestion. On the basis of experience with hundreds of patients, I am aware that there is much more to acupuncture than the power of suggestion alone. Yet at the same time I also recognize that this form of treatment is an excellent vehicle for suggestion.

The patient lies motionless on the table as needles are placed in various parts of his body. They soon produce unusual sensations and a feeling of relaxation. He is told this treatment will make him feel better, and can perceive for himself the very noticeable effects of the acupuncture. The somewhat exotic associations of acupuncture with an Eastern culture and a history stretching into the distant past also lend a certain element of mystery to the procedure.

I do not exaggerate this, yet I do not discourage it either. I see no reason not to make the fullest use of the power of suggestion available in acupuncture or any other treatment. It is not necessary to separate physiological changes produced by the treatment from those that are a result of the associated suggestion. The main purpose is to help the patient, regardless of precisely how this is accomplished.

The Ubiquitous Placebo Effect

Acupuncture and other unconventional therapies are not the only places where suggestion may play a part. Its role in orthodox medical practice is at least as important, although rarely recognized to its full extent. Every time a doctor prescribes a drug and describes its potential effects, he is employing suggestion and enlisting the power of the patient's belief. The influence of this belief on the outcome of treatment is commonly referred to as the "placebo effect." The more successful the physician is in suggesting a positive outcome, the stronger this effect will be.

The placebo effect is dramatically demonstrated by experiments in which people who believe they are receiving a drug are instead given an inert pill that contains no active ingredient. The placebo pill will often have an effect similar to the actual drug, as long as the patient thinks he is getting the real medication. This effect is so ubiquitous that any research must include what is called a "placebo control." One group of people receives the drug to be tested, while an equivalent "placebo control group" is given a placebo. The response of each group is then compared to distinguish the effects of the drug from those of the suggestion.

The placebo effect is especially powerful when relatively subjective symptoms such as pain or anxiety are involved, but it is by no means limited to these conditions. Virtually any of the body's functions can be influenced by supplying an effective suggestion. Yet despite the enormous capacity of suggestion to produce changes, its practical applications are neglected.

The capricious tendency of human beings to get well simply because they are told they will is more often viewed as an inconvenient complication of research design than as a potential source of healing. Suggestion introduces an unpredictable variable into a system that attempts to explain all observations in terms of purely physical cause and effect. From this perspective, everything would be a lot simpler if people only got better when they were given a real drug and there was no such thing as a placebo effect to complicate the matter.

Thus, the effects of suggestion tend to be ignored in actual practice. If researchers find no difference between a drug and a placebo control, they will conclude that the drug is worthless, but they will *not* arrive at the far more fascinating conclusion that suggestion in itself may be an effective form of treatment for whatever condition is being studied.

In medical practice, a half-humorous remark is sometimes made that a doctor had best use a new drug while it still works. Throughout medical history, various drugs or other treatments have been introduced and have enjoyed apparent success for a while, only to disappear from use. It would seem that these therapies worked as long as doctors and their patients believed in them, but then were abandoned when this belief was lost.

In the early part of this century, one treatment for *angina pectoris*—chest pain caused by a narrowing of the blood vessels to the heart—was the administration of ordinary bicarbonate of soda. Now that we have a greater understanding of how the chest pain of angina is produced, this treatment has been given up as worthless.

However, while it was in common use, many people experienced relief of their symptoms from this treatment. Because angina can be extensively influenced by emotional factors, it would seem that this relief was a product of the positive suggestion accompanying the treatment.

While we now realize that many past medical practices had no real effect other than suggestion, it is more difficult to view our current practices in the same light. Yet it is useful to remember that the eighteenth-century physician probably prescribed leeches for his patients as seriously as we now prescribe our favorite drugs—and that the mechanism of suggestion through which both produce results may be more similar than modern doctors would like to think.

Surgery and Suggestion

When we think of a placebo, we usually think of a pill. But a placebo effect may also be involved in other forms of treatment. Even in surgery, the branch of medicine that involves the most direct physical manipulation of the body, the role of suggstion may be important. If a doctor can produce positive results simply by prescribing some pills, how much stronger might the implicit suggestion be in a surgical procedure? The patient is put into deep sleep, and his body is actually cut open to correct or remove some malfunctioning part. He is then brought back to life and told that he is well. It would be hard to imagine a more symbolically impressive context for successful healing.

Most surgeons have a strong belief in the power of what they do, and it is not surprising that patients are attracted to surgeons who express great personal confidence. Although they may not think of it in such terms, these surgeons are making excellent use of the power of suggestion to encourage a positive outcome. Certainly the patient who approaches surgery with confidence in his doctor is more likely to do well.

Positive expectations can also be intentionally enhanced with direct suggestion. A number of times I have hypnotized patients specifically for this purpose. A day or two before surgery, they were given suggestions for a successful result, smooth awakening from anaesthesia, rapid healing, little postoperative pain, or anything else appropriate to their situation. All found this very reassuring, and reported later that everything went smoothly with their surgery. There is no reason why such simple preparation could not be incorporated more often into the preoperative routine.

There have even been reports in recent years that patients may be influenced by suggestions made to them *during* surgery, while under anaesthesia. It appears that the unconscious mind may be more aware of what is taking place in the anaesthetized state than we imagine. This presents the intriguing possibility that doctors could encourage a positive outcome for some patients by what they say during surgery. It also means that if anaesthetized patients are not really as oblivious to what is happening as they seem, then we should at least consider the idea of avoiding comments during surgery that could produce serious negative effects.

How Doctors Communicate with Patients

Communication skills should be a fundamental part of the medical school curriculum, taught along with other fundamentals such as anatomy or physiology. However, like most doctors, I was taught nothing about suggestion. Only as I began to practice medicine did I come to realize that I was able to influence people not only by what I did but by *how* I did it. I became fascinated by this aspect of medicine and was anxious to take the fullest advantage of it.

My first approach was very direct. I enthusiastically encouraged all my patients to expect that whatever we were doing would lead to positive results. This was simple and at times very successful. But at other times it led to problems, and I soon realized that this approach was somewhat naive.

Not everyone responded well to my suggestions, and those who did not were sometimes disappointed or upset. They felt, with some justification, that I had led them to expect unrealistic results. Obviously something else was needed in these situations. For some people, the simple statement that they will feel better is not a sufficiently sophisticated way to encourage a positive outcome.

It is also necessary to be realistic about the results that can actually be expected from any treatment. An overly optimistic prediction that is not fulfilled can destroy the doctor's future credibility with the patient. This risk can be avoided if the doctor provides positive suggestions more indirectly.

Suggestions can often be more effective when they are incorporated into conversation in an unobtrusive fashion. An expectation of positive results can be communicated "between the lines," by such things as the demeanor of the physician, his tone of voice, or the choice of wording in a phrase. Such indirect suggestion requires maintaining a sensitivity to what is going on between doctor and patient at each moment, and is really what much of the doctor's so-called "bedside manner" is all about.

Effective suggestions cannot be communicated by routine, but must be tailored to each individual situation. This is not always easy, and the physician is often challenged to sense just what note to strike with each patient. This skill cannot be taught in the same way as learning which drug to prescribe for a particular symptom. But, like any skill, it is governed by certain basic principles and can be developed with practice.

More than we may realize, we create our reality

through what we choose to believe. If you are convinced that you are sick and incapable of getting well, then it will be difficult for you to do so unless this belief is changed. On the other hand, if you are convinced that you *can* get well, then you have at least created the circumstances in which it is possible for this to happen. The more strongly you believe in this outcome, the more powerful a force the belief can be to actually bring it about.

The particular set of beliefs you hold is shaped by information from many sources. Inevitably, these beliefs are influenced by other people. What they say or do can affect what you think about your own health. And because of his unique position, the individual who can often exert the greatest influence is the physician.

This is a serious responsibility. It is also a great gift to be invested by others with such special influence. When used well, it can be a powerful force for healing. If, through my behavior, I can create a more positive set of beliefs in another person, then I have perhaps provided a more fundamental level of help than any specific treatment could offer.

8

Perspectives on Healing: East and West

The Life Energy of the Body

Modern Western medicine recognizes both the physical and psychological aspects of illness, but tends to keep them in separate compartments. A certain overlap *is* acknowledged, but these two categories remain essentially distinct fields of medicine. It is the doctor's job to treat physical illness, while emotional illness is left to the psychologist or psychiatrist.

We accept that physical problems can lead to emotional complaints, but the reverse is largely ignored. The possibility that something as tangible as physical disease can be created by "intangible" emotions is drastically underestimated. This distinction between mind and body results in fragmented medical care that may only partially address the cause of an illness.

Much of what is popularly called "holistic" medicine today is aimed at erasing this arbitrary separation and approaching illness as something that involves the *whole* person. Often this has involved exploring ideas that are not a part of conventional medicine, but may have their origins in other cultures. As both doctors and patients who are interested in such an approach search for a broader perspective on health and illness, they have turned especially to the ancient cultures of the East. Thus, concepts that originated in the distant past, and on the other side of the planet, are now finding their way into contemporary American medicine.

Among traditional medical practices of India, China, or Japan, we find not only different treatment techniques, but a different perspective on the human organism as well. Western medicine concerns itself primarily with the physical body, altering its condition through drugs or surgery. Traditional Eastern medicine also deals with the physical body, but recognizes as well a less tangible energy that underlies the physical condition. Thus, its approach to treatment may be in terms of manipulating this energy to bring about change on the physical level.

The concept of an underlying life energy helps avoid the arbitrary separation of mind and body. Instead, both physical and mental symptoms can be viewed as different manifestations of the same energy that reflect the condition of the whole person.

In traditional Chinese medicine, the body's energy is referred to as *chi* (*ki* in Japanese medicine), while in the Ayurvedic system of India it is called *prana*. All describe in similar terms an energy field that underlies the material body. Although it eludes precise definition, this energy is a manifestation within each individual of the universal energy that animates everything that is alive.

Harnessed on different levels, this energy is the force that allows the martial artist to break boards with his hands, the acupuncturist to heal with his needles, or the accomplished yogi to remain comfortably warm in freezing temperatures. While its existence is difficult to measure objectively, a subjective sense of its reality is available to anyone prepared to seriously observe the workings of his or her own body.

The field of energy is pictured as circulating throughout the body. In traditional Chinese medicine, specific pathways of energy flow are described that run lengthwise through the head, trunk, and extremities. Twelve major pathways are located on either side of the body, each of which corresponds in a complex fashion to one of the major organ systems. Two additional pathways follow along the midline of the body, one in front and one in back. Secondary pathways are connected to this primary system.

The continual movement of *chi* takes place along these pathways, and symptoms of illness are thought to result from some imbalance or blockage in this flow. Treatment, therefore, aims to correct the physical symptoms by adjusting this underlying imbalance. The idea of health as synonymous with balance is repeatedly encountered in Oriental medicine, and treatment is often described by elaborate metaphors of restoring harmonious function within the entire organism.

Health as Balance

The fundamental expression of balance is the classical symbol of *yin* and *yang*. The familiar image of the circle formed by two equal, complementary portions, each of which defines and merges with the other, represents the interaction of opposing principles that create a perfectly balanced whole. This concept, so simple, yet so rich in its complexity, permeates Oriental philosophy and applies equally to events within the body and in the world. In worldly phenomena we see the interaction of light and darkness, heat and cold, male and female, as well as many other opposing forces. All can be described as manifestations of *yin* and *yang*.

These same principles have their equivalents within the body, where opposing energies must remain in balance for a state of health to exist. Although often obscured, Western medicine also recognizes this concept of balance in its description of the body. For example, move-

ment never involves only a single muscle, but is produced
by the graceful interplay of opposing muscles. One muscle group flexes the arm, while another straightens it, and
neither can work properly without the other. If, for any
reason, one of these opposing muscles ceases to function,
then normal movement will no longer be possible.

Similar phenomena are also found on a cellular level.
The nervous system, for example, functions through the
interaction of opposing impulses of electrical excitation
and inhibition. Through the constantly changing balance
of these opposites, activity in the nervous system reaches
an extraordinary level of complexity. Without the presence of both opposing forces, the nervous system would
cease to function.

And influencing every part of the body, we have the
autonomic nervous system, whose two divisions—the
sympathetic and parasympathetic—are so constructed
that all their actions oppose and balance one another. One
increases the heart rate and blood pressure, while the
other lowers them; one stimulates the process of digestion, the other slows it down; one dilates the pupil of the
eye, the other causes it to constrict. The list goes on at
great length and includes all activities not normally under
conscious control.

The relative predominance of either division varies as
the body adapts to changing circumstances. When immediate physical action is required, for example, the sympathetic division takes control, while the parasympathetic
assumes a more dominant role as you relax after a heavy
meal. Each situation we encounter requires a somewhat
different adjustment of the autonomic nervous system.

In a state of health, the opposing actions of the two
divisions blend smoothly, as the balance between them
shifts in response to changing events. Western medicine
refers to this process as "homeostasis." Yet this Western
term is really another way of describing what Chinese
medicine calls the balance of *yin* and *yang*. All we need do

is substitute the words yin and yang for "sympathetic" and "parasympathetic" to see these terms are describing the same thing.

The autonomic nervous system responds to both external influences and internal emotional states, and many illnesses can be considered the result of its dysfunction. Conceivably, Oriental techniques described to correct an imbalance of *yin* and *yang* might also be thought of as ways of balancing the autonomic nervous system. When put in these terms, the idea of treating *yin* and *yang* through stimulation of the body's energy pathways no longer seems so strange.

The *Chakras* and Life Energy

Ayurveda, the traditional medical system of India, has a concept of a field of energy similar to that found in Oriental medicine. However, here a more elaborate system of energy pathways is described, consisting of thousands of channels throughout the body, all of which are connected to a central channel along the spine. Along this central channel are located the seven major energy centers or *chakras*.

The Sanskrit word *chakra* means wheel, and represents what is described as a spinning wheel of energy. Each of the seven *chakras* represents a different aspect of the organism's functioning. They correspond in some respect to the major nerve centers located along the spine that are familiar to Western medicine. However, they have more significance than this purely physical correspondence, and can be understood psychologically and symbolically as well.

The most comprehensible description of the *chakras* that I have found is in the excellent book *Yoga and Psychotherapy*, written by Swami Rama and his associates at the Himalayan International Institute. They describe the *chakras* as centers where the relationship can be seen between "certain aspects of the physical world, the energy system, the mind and higher consciousness. For example, at the solar plexus, aggression, assertiveness, fire, heat, digestion, assimilation and active metabolism, intermix in a way that cuts across our separate concepts of what is physical, what is physiological and what is psychological."[1]

And again: "Each of the *chakras* has a rich meaning and is vast in its significance. Each center pulls together different aspects of the external and inner worlds into a coordinated, but difficult to describe, whole."[2]

The system of *chakras* provides a unified way to understand how certain physical and psychological events in the body may be related to each other. In a previous chapter, the connection between low back pain and certain emotional states was examined. In the context of Western medicine, it is not clear why such a relationship should exist, or what its significance might be. Thus, little is made of this correspondence other than to observe its existence. However, a relationship between physical and emotional events is inevitable according to the system of *chakras*.

In very simplified terms, events in the life of an individual may lead to a disturbance of particular energy centers—in the case of low back pain, the two lowest *chakras*—which is expressed by both physical and emotional symptoms characteristic of these centers. The patient experiences pain in the low back region, along with feelings of depression, insecurity, and diminished sexual activity.

The association of these various symptoms will be apparent to an observant physician. The concept of energy centers simply provides a coherent framework for considering the nature of this association. Rather than treating a patient for mechanical low back pain, anxiety/depression, and sexual dysfunction as separate problems that may even require different therapists, it is now possible to approach all of these conditions as manifestations of the same underlying state, and to treat the patient in a more unified way. This means not only prescribing muscle relaxants or antidepressants but addressing whatever factors precipitated the entire disturbance.

A skeptical Westerner might ask whether there really are such things as *chakras*, or whether they are only interesting metaphors for our experience. From a purely materialistic perspective, *chakras* might be considered no more than a fanciful interpretation of particular nerve centers in the body. Yet the question cannot really be answered only on this level. On a strictly physical level, the *chakras* are perhaps the same as nerve centers and the functions they control. But we do not exist on a purely physical level; we live psychologically and symbolically as well. The concept of *chakras* provides a way to become aware of the correspondences among these different levels of existence.

Although the systems of energy described in Ayurvedic or Oriental medicine have no equivalent in our own medical system, we do recognize the existence of electromagnetic fields. We even measure various forms of electrical activity to investigate what is taking place in the body. We perform electroencephalograms (EEGs) to measure electrical activity of the brain, electrocardiograms (EKGs) for the heart, and electromyograms (EMGs) to examine nerves and muscles.

We tend to imagine this electrical energy as a by-product of the material body—as though the body generates a field of energy through its functioning. However, it is possible to reverse this idea and claim that the presence of an energy field generates a physical body. Although this is foreign to our usual way of thinking, it is, in at least one sense, a more realistic description. At the moment of death, it is the energy field that ceases to exist, not the physical body. Thus it is not so much that the body generates an energy field, as that this energy is what gives life to the body.

We think of the physical body as solid and relatively unchanging, but this is something of an illusion. Our bodies undergo a slow and invisible process of constant repair and renewal; it is estimated that every cell is replaced within a span of seven years. Although you may appear the same when you look in the mirror in the morning, nearly every molecule of your body may be different from those present a few years ago.

If bodies undergo such transformation, the intriguing question arises of just what provides continuity in the life of the individual. The raw materials may change, yet some pattern or template exists upon which the physical body continues to be maintained in approximately the same form. On a physical level, Western medicine explains this by the existence of information coded in the DNA present in each cell. But from the perspective of Eastern medicine, this pattern is provided by the field of energy underlying the body.

Pursuing this line of thinking leads to some interesting consequences. If the body is forever in the process of replacing its physical substance, then perhaps some aspects of its condition are less fixed and more amenable to change than we may realize. By altering the underlying pattern of energy, perhaps the physical body has the potential to be altered in unexpected ways. This may also offer an explanation for situations in which patients unexpectedly recover from illness, despite the predictions of Western medicine to the contrary.

Wilhelm Reich and Orgone Energy

The concept of a basic life energy, as described in the medical traditions of the East, is not entirely new to our own culture. Earlier in this century, a similar idea was advanced in particularly dramatic fashion by Wilhelm Reich. Working from a purely Western background as a physician and psychiatrist, and with no apparent exposure to Eastern thought, his description of this life energy sounds remarkably similar to the Oriental concept of *chi*.

Reich was a highly original thinker whose concepts hovered between madness and genius, and many of his ideas were met with an extraordinarily hostile reception. Although his work is readily available today, it is incredible to realize that only thirty years ago in America his books were actually destroyed by agents of the federal government. In 1954, Reich himself was imprisoned for ignoring the prohibition of his work, and three years later he died in prison. However, today his books are once again in bookstores and libraries, and have helped provide the foundation for many unconventional therapies that are becoming increasingly popular in this country.

Reich called the life force he believed he had discovered "orgone energy." As in traditional Chinese medicine, his theory was that a free flow of this energy was necessary for health, and any blockage would result in illness. He further believed that such blockage was the result of what he called "muscular armoring," a chronic tension in the body that was the physical counterpart of repressed emotions.

Today this is not an entirely unfamiliar idea. But when first advanced by Reich, it represented what he considered an original way of understanding the condition of the body. According to Reich, muscular armoring always existed perpendicularly to the flow of energy, which, as in Oriental medicine, he saw moving lengthwise through the body. Most interestingly, he observed specific patterns of blockage that would occur repeatedly, and divided the body into seven discrete segments. The topmost, or "ocular" segment, consists of the forehead, eyes, and cheekbone area, and Reich's own description gives a feeling for what is meant by body armoring:

> In the sphere of the ocular armor segment, we find
> a contraction and immobilization of all or almost all

the muscles of the eyeballs, the eyelids, the forehead, the lachrymal gland, etc. Rigid forehead and eyelids, expressionless eyes or bulging eyeballs, mask-like expression, and immobility on both sides of the nose are the essential characteristics of this armor ring. The eyes peep out as from a rigid mask. . . . The forehead is without expression, as if it had been 'flattened out.' Nearsightedness, astigmatism, etc. very often exist.[3]

The remaining six segments are described as the "oral, neck, chest, diaphragmatic, abdominal and pelvic" segments. Blockages similar to that described for the first segment can also exist in any or all of these other segments. A disturbance at each of them is associated with its own characteristic physical and emotional expression. Only when all of these blockages are removed can the life energy flow freely, and the individual experience complete health.

This idea is again reminiscent of Eastern concepts of *chi* or *prana* in the body, but Reich went somewhat further. He postulated that the movement of energy in the body followed a rhythmic pattern: first, the accumulation of tension, followed by periodic discharge, and then relaxation. This pattern could be observed in the movements of all living creatures, from primitive invertebrates to man. But he believed that its most powerful expression in human beings occurred in the experience of total orgasm (from which Reich derived his term "orgone energy"). However, by this he meant not simply sexual release, but a profound discharge of energy involving the entire organism.

According to Reich, blockages among people in modern society made such free discharge of the body's energy impossible. He described the consequence of this not only as localized muscle tension, but the eventual development of illness in the area of the body where blockages existed. Reich was particularly interested in the idea that cancer could be a long-term consequence of such energy blockage. It was when he attempted to treat cancer patients with a device he claimed could concentrate orgone energy from the atmosphere that his work was halted and he was placed in prison.

From the viewpoint of conventional Western medicine, Reich's work is nothing more than outright quackery. Yet in light of the growing influence of non-Western thought in our culture, his ideas no longer seem quite so strange. There is a particularly striking equivalence between Reich's segmental division of the body and the classical description of the *chakra* system.

The seven major *chakras*, located along the spinal axis of the body, correspond remarkably well to Reich's seven segments of the body. And his description of specific physical and emotional patterns, associated with blockage at each level, fits perfectly with the idea that a disturbance at each of the *chakras* has characteristic symptoms. It is especially interesting that Reich apparently had no familiarity with the idea of *chakras*, but arrived at a similar description from personal observations.

Repressed Emotions and Illness

Regardless of what one thinks of his more extraordinary theories, it is at least apparent to any careful observer that Reich's descriptions of "muscular armor" reflect a very sharp clinical eye. I find myself nodding in agreement as I read them, for the patterns he describes so vividly occur repeatedly in the patients who pass through my office. The following is his description of muscular armoring involving the fourth, or chest segment, a frequently observed condition:

The armoring of the chest is manifested in the elevation of the bony structure, a chronic attitude of inhalation, shallow breathing, and immobility of the thorax. We already know that the attitude of inhalation is the most important instrument in the suppression of *any* kind of emotion. . . . All the intercostal muscles, the large chest muscles (pectoral), the shoulder muscles (deltoid), and the muscle group on and between the shoulder blades are involved in the armoring of the chest. . . . Shoulders which are pulled back express precisely what they mean—'holding back.' . . . Most of the emotional expressive movements of the arms and hands also stem from the plasmatic emotions of the organs of the chest. . . . The inhibition of the inner chest organs usually entails an inhibition of those arm movements which express 'desire,' 'embracing,' or 'reaching for something.'[4]

This presentation of the relationship between blocked emotions and chronic muscle tension is relevant for any physician. It is not an abstract theory, but a clear description of patterns that can be observed consistently in the bodies of real people. The possible relationship of these patterns to illness is somewhat more controversial.

It is not entirely unreasonable to assume that chronic muscular blockage could ultimately lead to more serious illness in that part of the body. Nerves and blood vessels are located in the muscles and connective tissues, so it would not be surprising for their activity to be affected in some way by the condition of these tissues. Further, because nerves and blood vessels nourish and regulate the internal organs, anything affecting their functioning could create a predisposition toward dysfunction in the organs as well. And if this condition persisted over a prolonged period of time, it might ultimately lead to the appearance of significant illness.

This line of reasoning encourages intriguing speculation about the origins of illness. For example, could chronic muscle tension and associated blockage of energy in
the chest be connected in some way with a predisposition
to heart disease? A Western physician might scoff at this
possibility, yet we know that a tendency toward heart
disease is associated with certain types of personality, just
as muscle armoring in the chest is associated with particular emotional states.

It is possible that this muscular condition could alter
the flow of vital energy to the associated organs. Although
this energy is difficult to define exactly, it includes elements that correspond to the breath, the circulation of the
blood, and the activity of the nerves—all essential factors
in determining the health of various organs.

We could speculate even further about the condition of
the body's muscular structure and other forms of illness.
An interesting example is chronic pelvic inflammation in
women, a condition that has become very common in
recent years.

Although various theories propose new micro-
organisms involved in this disorder, it is still difficult to
explain why it occurs so frequently today. Usually it is
treated with antibiotics. Sometimes this works, but at
other times it achieves only limited results. Women with
this problem often experience recurrent episodes of pelvic pain and receive repeated courses of different antibiotics in an attempt to control the symptoms.

However, it is also possible to look at this problem in
terms of blockage in the pelvic region. Although it is
difficult to generalize, I have a sense that many women I
have seen with unexplained pelvic inflammatory disease
also experience greater-than-average sexual conflict or
dysfunction in their lives. This is the sort of correlation
that cannot be confirmed by formal scientific measurement. Yet it is an observation that I have heard from other

physicians who see such patients. If it is true, then it could provide an explanation for increased muscular armoring in the pelvic region. Thus, this illness might be thought of not only as an infection to be treated with antibiotics, but also as a problem of chronic pelvic tension related to emotional stress.

Many other medical problems also lend themselves to such speculation. Could the eventual appearance of arthritis in a joint have any relationship to chronic rigidity in that part of the body? Or could conditions favorable for the development of a tumor be created by subtle alterations in blood flow and nervous activity caused by chronic muscle tension over a period of time? This idea is different from the biochemical perspective usually taken by Western medicine, yet the two approaches are not mutually exclusive. Chronic blockage of energy flow may set the stage for the biochemical events associated with specific illness.

The theory of an energy field underlying the physical body broadens our concept of what the human organism is and how it works. For anyone concerned with health care, it provides another way of looking at illness that opens up new approaches to treatment.

NOTES

1. Swami Rama, Rudolph Ballentine M.D., and Swami Ajaya (Allan Weinstock Ph.D.), *Yoga and Psychotherapy* (Honesdale, PA: Himalayan International Institute of Yoga Science and Philosophy, 1976), p. 221.

2. Ibid., p. 225.

3. Wilhelm Reich, *Selected Writings: An Introduction to Orgonomy* (New York: Farrar, Straus & Giroux, 1951), p. 153.

4. Ibid., p. 157.

9

Acupuncture and
Western Medicine

Acupuncture in America

The concepts of Oriental medicine have given rise to
forms of treatment different from those used in the West.
One of these is acupuncture. Not many years ago, there
was scarcely a person in America who had ever heard of
acupuncture. But in the early 1970s, Westerners once
again began to visit China and they brought back reports
of an unusual form of medicine practiced there. It involved the stimulation of various points on the surface of
the body by the insertion of small needles.

For those accustomed to Western medicine, this
seemed most unusual, but many stories described medical conditions successfully treated with acupuncture.
Most remarkable were the reports of its use in surgery.
With the insertion of a few strategically placed needles,
patients in China were undergoing major surgery without general anaesthesia, and apparently feeling no pain,
although they were fully awake.

While this was all new to America, it was by no means
a new development in China. Although the origins of
acupuncture have been lost in time, we know this treatment has been practiced continuously in China for at

least three thousand years. Considering the enormous political and cultural changes that have occurred in China during this time, acupuncture has shown remarkable endurance. We think of it as something unusual, yet it is quite possible that more people have been treated with acupuncture than with any other formalized system of medicine in human history.

The news stories about acupuncture in the early 1970s reached me at an opportune time. I was beginning to investigate alternatives to standard Western medical practice, and acupuncture seemed to represent an entirely new approach to treatment. If people really were being treated successfully with acupuncture, as well as undergoing surgery without anaesthesia, then there were important aspects of the human body not known to Western medicine.

I was determined to learn something about acupuncture, but at that time, and even today, there were no formal training programs for physicians, so individual doctors had to make their own arrangements. Eventually I joined a group at the UCLA School of Medicine that was conducting research in acupuncture as well as treating patients. We saw as many as two hundred patients a week at our acupuncture clinic, many with chronic pain problems, though a variety of other conditions were presented as well. The results were impressive. Although many of our patients came with difficult problems, and were trying acupuncture as a last resort after conventional therapy had failed to help, they frequently had a good response.

The Experience of Acupuncture

I became further intrigued by acupuncture when I had the opportunity to experience it myself. As part of an acupuncture research project, I was naturally interested in knowing what it was like to receive a treatment. However, like many other people, I had a definite dislike for "needles," and I viewed the insertion of several acupuncture needles at once with misgivings.

Fortunately, as I have long since learned, needle placement can be essentially painless, and I felt very little sensation as the needles were inserted in my skin. Acupuncture needles are actually like fine, flexible pins made of stainless steel, and, unlike the familiar Western needles used for injections or to draw blood, they are not hollow. Thus, they do not tear the skin, but slide in smoothly and rarely leave even a mark after they are removed.

I laid down on the treatment table and placed myself in the hands of the acupuncturist. He swabbed a bit of alcohol on several spots and then quickly and deftly inserted needles in these places. When each needle reached the proper depth, it produced the characteristic feeling so familiar to anyone who receives acupuncture. I felt a sensation similar to a dull aching or tingling where the first needle was placed in the back of my hand. This soon progressed to a feeling of heaviness and mild numbness in my entire arm.

Other needles placed elsewhere produced similar sensations, and soon a numb, slightly giddy feeling seemed to pervade my entire body. My arms and legs felt heavy, as though they would be difficult to move. The sensations hovered oddly on the edge between pleasure and pain— the entire experience was mildly uncomfortable yet pleasurable at the same time.

I remained on the table with eight needles in various parts of my body for about twenty minutes. During this time, the sensations at each point were occasionally intensified by brief, gentle manipulation of the needles. Traditional acupuncturists refer to these sensations as a sign that the *chi,* or life energy, of the body is being stimulated. In fact, this describes very well how I felt. I experienced what I could call a flow or movement of

energy in my body. While difficult to convey in words, it
was clear to me in a way that no amount of theories read in
books could ever be that this acupuncture had done *something* to my body.

Following the treatment, I felt quite relaxed and at
ease in my body for the remainder of the day. I have since
observed this to be a typical response among those who
receive acupuncture. It is not uncommon to fall into a
deep, restful sleep later in the day or that night, or to
experience a mild euphoria or "spaced-out" feeling. The
extent of this reaction varies; for some it is a sense of mild
relaxation, while for others it may involve a powerful
release of tension.

There are several hundred acupuncture points, each
of which can be precisely located by reference to specific
anatomical features. The choice of just which of these to
use is determined by many factors, including the characteristics of the individual patient, the nature of the illness,
and a complex set of interrelationships that exist among
the pathways on which the points lie. These points have a
definite physical reality, and many are well known in
other disciplines. Acupuncture points are commonly
used, for example, as pressure points in massage and in
the martial arts.

Acupuncture points have also been independently described by Western scientists investigating the electrical
properties of muscles. Within each muscle in the body is a
specific point that has the lowest threshold to electrical
stimulation. These points are known in Western medicine as "motor points," and they have the same anatomical location in all individuals. What is interesting is that
nearly all of these points seem to be identical with acupuncture points, so much so that a textbook illustration of
motor points will appear quite recognizable to anyone
familiar with acupuncture.

Acupuncture points also possess the intriguing but as
yet unexplained property of decreased electrical re-

sistance compared to surrounding areas on the skin. Thus it is actually possible to locate many points with an electrical probe that measures fine variations in resistance. In practice, however, a serious acupuncturist would not need such help. A skilled examiner can locate acupuncture points by sensing a subtle depression in the tissues or a greater sensitivity to pressure, as well as by the relation of the points to anatomical landmarks.

Acupuncture points are not an abstraction of Oriental philosophy; they are quite real and have an anatomically consistent location in everyone. However, it is less clear how these hundreds of points are connected with each other. According to traditional theory, they mark the places where the body's energy flow is accessible to stimulation. In any acupuncture textbook the energy pathways, or "meridians," on which the points lie will be boldly illustrated, as they have been described for thousands of years. Yet unlike the points themselves, the meridians have no equivalence in any modern scientific system.

Perhaps the meridians represent some aspect of the nervous system understood by a sophisticated, ancient civilization but unknown to modern science. Or perhaps they simply represent an entirely different perspective on the functioning of the body. The metaphor that appeals to me most is the acupuncture system as a sort of map on the surface of the body to some part of the neuro-endocrine system. The more skillful one is at reading this map, the greater the possibilities for influencing what occurs in the body through stimulation of appropriate points.

New Theories of Acupuncture

Much of the investigation of acupuncture in the West has been aimed at describing it in terms comprehensible to our culture. Because acupuncture has gained most acceptance here as a treatment for pain, this is the area where most research has been done.

How can sticking small needles in various parts of the body lead to successful relief of pain? Some theories have suggested that stimulation of acupuncture points can generate impulses in nerves, that, at some level of the nervous system, interfere with other impulses involved in the transmission of pain. These theories offer a partial explanation for certain observations about acupuncture, but none so far have been able to explain it completely. However, they do a least provide a beginning for thinking about acupuncture in Western terms.

The newest explanation of how acupuncture relieves pain arose from the recent discovery of endorphins. The term "endorphin," a contraction of the words "endogenous morphine," refers to substances present in small amounts in the nervous system. Endorphins are capable of a powerful pain-relieving effect, identical to that of morphine but many times greater.

The discovery that human beings actually produce such a substance in their bodies has generated much interest in scientific circles. It has also captured the imagination of the media, which has made endorphin almost a household word in only a few years. The idea that certain kinds of exercise, for example, may stimulate production of endorphins has been offered as an explanation for such things as "runner's high," the feeling of exhilaration described after prolonged running or other forms of exercise. The role of endorphins in the body's biochemistry has been widely investigated, and we now know they are not a single substance, but a number of different, closely related compounds, each with specific properties.

The relevance of endorphins to acupuncture is demonstrated by the interesting observation that the pain-relieving effects of acupuncture can apparently be blocked by certain drugs. These drugs are narcotic antagonists, commonly used to treat overdoses of narcotics. They interfere with the action of morphine or other narcotics, and, similarly, also interfere with the action of endorphins. Thus, if narcotic antagonists also interfere with the effects of acupuncture, this suggests that acupuncture may relieve pain by stimulating the body to produce endorphins. Although this remains only a theory, present evidence seems to point in this direction.

Other properties of endorphins also lead to intriguing speculation about acupuncture. It seems that endorphins not only relieve pain, they exert other powerful effects on the body. Certain endorphins have the capacity to alter psychological states, while others seem to act upon basic regulatory mechanisms such as maintenance of body temperature.

It seems likely that as endorphins continue to be investigated, more and more substances will be found that are capable of affecting a wide range of human behavior and functioning. It is interesting to speculate that stimulation of various acupuncture points can lead to the release in the body of a variety of endorphins or similar substances not yet identified. Perhaps the accomplished acupuncturist, although describing what he does in very different terms, is actually orchestrating the release of tiny amounts of potent substances in the nervous system to produce a variety of effects upon the patient.

Whether we talk about acupuncture in terms of the flow of *chi* or the release of endorphins, the difference is essentially one of words. However, the theory of endorphins seems to have given acupuncture greater credibility in the eyes of Western science. Doctors are used to thinking in terms of drugs, and the discovery of endorphins provides a drug of sorts to explain the effects of acupuncture—but in this case it is a drug produced by the patient himself.

Recently I was talking with a patient about acupuncture and describing what it would involve. After I had finished my explanation, she turned to me with a somewhat puzzled look and asked: "What's in those needles anyway that's going to help me?" This is a question I have been asked before by other patients. In America, we associate being stuck with a needle with injection of a drug. The patient still looked a bit dubious after I explained there was nothing in the needles and that whatever was going to help her was within her own body.

The fact that acupuncture does not involve any external agent, but acts by stimulating some intrinsic function of the body, whether we call it *chi* or endorphins, suggests both its advantages and limitations. Because it acts upon the body's own mechanisms of self-regulation, acupuncture is unlikely to worsen existing problems. Though it may sometimes be ineffective, I have never seen a patient experience any long-term ill effects from acupuncture. As I often tell potential patients, the worst that can happen is that nothing will happen. At a time when we are seeing so many serious problems from the side effects of drug therapy, this is a significant advantage for any treatment.

This same property also imposes certain limits to what can be expected from acupuncture, because the response to treatment will be determined by the internal capacity of each individual. In practical terms, this means that chronically ill or debilitated patients—or those who have mistreated their bodies with poor diet, excessive alcohol, or other destructive habits—may not respond as quickly as those in better health. Yet even in the presence of serious illness, powerful reserves of life force may still be tapped. I can sometimes recognize which people are more likely to respond to acupuncture, although I can never predict this with certainty. Sometimes the results of treatment are even a surprise to me as the doctor.

A Remarkable Recovery

I once received a telephone call from a rather distraught older woman, Mrs. Butler, asking for my help. She told me that her husband was too weak to make the trip to my office, and asked if I could please come to their home to treat him with acupuncture. I do not usually make calls at home, but she sounded so anxious that I agreed to come the following morning. Her husband was an eighty-year-old man who, several months previously, had been stricken with an unexplained illness that had left him unable to swallow. His doctors suspected some unusual viral illness was responsible, but had been unable to make a diagnosis with any certainty or figure out how to help him.

For several months, Mr. Butler had been fed using a tube inserted through his nose to his stomach, but he was now growing unable to tolerate this any longer. After each meal, he would experience severe nausea and vomiting, and was gradually becoming thinner and weaker from his inability to retain food. He was also growing increasingly depressed about his condition. Medications no longer seemed to help the nausea, and his doctors could not tell him when, if ever, his ability to swallow would return. As a last resort, his wife had decided to see if acupuncture might relieve his nausea.

When I arrived at their home the next day, I could see why Mr. Butler had not wanted to travel to my office. He had apparently been a healthy, alert man until a few months ago, but his prolonged illness was gradually wearing him down. His muscles were wasted, he moved very slowly, and he was at times confused about recent events. I told his wife that I would do my best, but that I really did not know how much I would be able to help. As I treated Mr. Butler, he lay quietly and scarcely seemed to notice the insertion of the needles, and I did not feel especially optimistic about his response. After I had finished, I asked his wife to call me the next day to report on how he was doing.

When she phoned the next day, I was amazed to hear happiness and excitement in her voice. She told me her husband had experienced absolutely no nausea since the treatment, and for the first time in a long while had been able to take a good deal of food. But even more remarkable was the change in his behavior. After spending the last few days in bed, he had gotten up and dressed himself, and for the first time since his illness began, he had sat down and played the piano.

His wife was very impressed with this remarkable change and so was I. It was really more than either of us had even dared to expect. Mr. Butler had appreciated my willingness to come to his home, and there was certainly an element of positive suggestion in what took place between us. But there was clearly more involved here. The stimulation of appropriate acupuncture points had led to definite physiological changes in his body that were reflected both physically and emotionally.

A few days later, Mr. Butler felt well enough to come to my office for his next treatment. I continued to see him regularly for several months, during which time his nausea was kept under control with acupuncture. He was again able to take food through his feeding tube and gradually he gained weight and grew stonger. During the course of treatment, I also began to select acupuncture points that I thought might stimulate his ability to swallow. I told him honestly that I had no idea whether this would help, but that it was worth a try.

For several weeks there was no change at all, but then slowly it seemed that his ability to swallow was beginning to return. By now, his nausea was no longer a problem and I did not need to see him regularly. Then one day after not seeing him for some time, he entered my office with a big smile on his face and the feeding tube gone. To the surprise of his doctors, who had predicted only a small chance of recovery, his swallowing had completely returned to normal.

It is impossible to determine how much acupuncture played a role in his recovery and how much it was simply the natural course of an unusual and poorly understood illness. It is also difficult to know how much my suggestion that I was doing something helpful influenced the outcome. Nevertheless, Mr. Butler is convinced that acupuncture was the stimulus to his dramatic recovery, and I cannot help but feel that it must have played an important part. A case like Mr. Butler's gives me great satisfaction. However, it also tantalizes me with the possibilities of acupuncture that I know must exist but that I am not always able to utilize so successfully.

Another patient with an extraordinary response to acupuncture was Mr. Richards. He was a forty-two-year-old truck driver who had complained of low back pain for several years following an automobile accident. He had seen several different doctors during this time, but had received no help for his problem other than prescriptions for various pain pills. Now he had decided he would like to try acupuncture. I agreed to treat him, but explained that the results would be difficult to predict. I also told him we would probably need to do a number of treatments, as he had already had this problem for several years.

Mr. Richards lay down on the treatment table, and shortly after the needles were inserted told me that he "felt something release" in his back. When the treatment was finished, he got up and stretched and told me that his back felt a lot looser. I asked him to come back a week later for his next treatment, and when he returned he told me that his pain was gone. It was not just better—it was gone completely. It had disappeared the day of his treatment and had not returned.

We were both amazed at such an immediate response in a condition that had been present for years. I even felt a bit foolish at having accomplished this dramatic cure without quite knowing how I had done it. In any event, there was no need for more treatment if he no longer had any pain, and I simply asked him to return if the pain should recur. He never did. Occasionally I would pass him in the street and he would continue to assure me that his back remained fine.

I cannot explain exactly what happened with Mr. Richards, or why the same thing does not happen with all the people I see with low back pain. His description of feeling something release in his back is suggestive of the traditional Oriental concept of chronic pain as a form of blocked energy that must be released, and perhaps in his case, this is the most appropriate way of understanding what occurred.

From time to time, just the right interaction occurs between doctor and patient, and acupuncture leads to remarkable results. I am convinced it is not merely a matter of effective suggestion. I have seen enough skeptical patients dragged into my office by someone else to try acupuncture who have still done extremely well. My best explanation is that when acupuncture is dramatically successful, it is because the organism is somehow prepared for the process of healing to take place, which is then triggered by the appropriate stimulus.

The Limits of Acupuncture

When acupuncture is not successful, it may be that the individual's healing capacity is simply unequal to the task of getting well, no matter how much this capacity is stimulated. This is sometimes the case for older patients whose symptoms may have been present for twenty years or more by the time they are seen for treatment. There are also situations in which something more than acupuncture is needed. This is particularly true when emotional problems underlie the physical symptoms.

One of the most common complaints among patients in my practice involves the constellation of symptoms arising from pain and tension in the neck and shoulder muscles. These symptoms are sometimes triggered by injury and are almost invariably worsened by stress. A vicious cycle of pain and muscle spasm can become established, with each reinforcing the other until the condition becomes chronic and difficult to relieve. Acupuncture can help to interrupt this cycle, but the basic problem may remain unresolved until the patient can recognize and deal with its cause.

Joan was an attractive and intelligent woman of twenty-seven who complained of severe pain in her neck and shoulders. It had reached the point where even simple movements of her head caused discomfort. She had heard that acupuncture might help and was anxious to try anything that could provide some relief. As we talked, I learned that she had lived with a man for several years but for a long time now had thought of leaving him. She was dissatisfied with their relationship, yet she feared the pain that a separation would mean. In her mind, she had repeatedly vacillated between leaving or staying.

More than anything, the ambivalence of her situation was difficult for her. The stress of her continued internal dialogue was reflected in the tightness of her neck and shoulder muscles. I sensed waves of tension radiating from her, filling the room, and I had to make a particular effort not to take on her tension myself.

As she lay on the table with the acupuncture needles in place, she gradually began to relax. By the end of the treatment, there was an easing of the discomfort in her movements and her speech, but the deep knot of tension inside her was still there. Afterward, we talked about the connection between her physical pain and her need to somehow resolve her situation. When she left the office, she made another appointment for the following week.

At the last moment Joan called to cancel her next visit. Twice more she scheduled appointments, only to cancel them with various excuses. I sensed she did not want to return because she had not made any real change in her situation.

Finally she did come back, and indeed there had been no change. Her neck was a little better than before, and again there was some relief after acupuncture, but the treatment still had not penetrated to the heart of her tension. This time she did not schedule another appointent, but told me she would call when she wanted to come again, and we both realized that further help would really have to come from within herself. Some weeks later I passed her on the street. She told me she was now living alone and her pain was gone.

For Joan, acupuncture had partly relieved her physical symptoms. The relaxation it provided had probably also helped her in the process of making a difficult personal decision. But acupuncture alone could not solve her problem. It could not remove her symptoms completely until she faced the underlying reason for their presence.

In this sense, the application of needles, by itself, is no different from taking medication in a pill. Both provide relief of symptoms. The advantage of acupuncture is that it involves none of the problems associated with medications, but is a technique for stimulating the body's *own* mechanism of self-regulation to operate more effectively.

Acupuncture also seems to operate on a level that may transcend the arbitrary distinction between physical and psychological symptoms. It often leads not only to relief of specific physical symptoms, but to a more intangible lightening of the spirit as well. The patient simply feels better in an overall way that is difficult to define precisely but is nevertheless quite real.

Any doctor sees many patients like Joan. Their physical pain is related to what is happening in their lives, and is accompanied by feelings of anxiety or depression, or often both. Acupuncture alone, or any other treatment directed solely at relieving symptoms, may be insufficient to resolve their problem. But it can still provide valuable help while one seeks some resolution of the underlying source of the symptoms.

Eastern and Western Medicine Combined

Although he may offer other treatment along with it, a traditional acupuncturist will consider acupuncture not only a useful technique, but a system of medicine that is complete in itself. In China today, traditional doctors treat everything from the common cold to appendicitis to schizophrenia with acupuncture. Because acupuncture acts by somehow normalizing the functioning of the body, it could potentially help relieve nearly any sort of medical problem, but there are some conditions for which it is clearly more appropriate than others.

As mentioned earlier, acupuncture treatment has had most acceptance in America for pain-related problems. In my practice I see many people with low back pain, neck and shoulder pain, arthritis, bursitis, migraine and tension headaches, and other conditions involving chronic pain. However, I have also had success in using acupuncture for many other problems. Patients with asthma, allergies, ringing in the ears, menstrual irregularities, colitis, chronic bronchitis, digestive disorders—to mention just a few examples—have all received effective treatment.

Acupuncture is also employed as an aid in controlling addictive or compulsive behavior involving drugs, cigarettes, or food. I may also use it in situations where no clear diagnosis can be made, but the patient continues to complain of just not feeling quite right. Often the acupuncture helps to snap a patient out of this state and stimulates a return to normal.

When I treat a patient with acupuncture, I rely to a certain extent upon general rules and information in textbooks, but also upon my own intuitive sense. Thus, I cannot always logically explain why I choose one set of acupuncture points rather than another for a given treatment. This is in contrast to Western medicine, where two well-trained physicians will ideally choose precisely the same course of action.

However, while I appreciate the more intuitive aspect of patient care, I would certainly not wish to discard Western medical science. Fortunately, it is not necessary to choose between one or the other. Acupuncture provides an alternative system for describing the condition of the body, and though it is different, it is not necessarily incorrect or imaginary. Conversely, accepting the reality of acupuncture does not mean we have to reject our own medical system. It is possible for these two very different descriptions to be accepted as real and valid. Both provide a true picture, seen from different perspectives. And these perspectives can be complementary to each other.

A familiarity with both Western and Eastern medicine allows one to see the body from a vantage not possible with either of them alone. By looking simultaneously from two perspectives, a new dimension emerges. Vision with either eye alone is flat and two dimensional, yet when both eyes are open at once, the images spring into three-dimensional depth.

When I examine a patient, I observe the various organs and parts of the body in Western terms. I can think in these terms and arrive at a diagnosis within this framework. Yet I am also aware of a network of acupuncture points and energy pathways superimposed upon this, so I can also think in these terms. At times, what is happening in the body can best be understood in terms of the flow and balance of life energy. At other times, a clearer picture is provided by a Western diagnosis of the physical condition.

Even if I were never to practice acupuncture again, my awareness of the additional perspective it provides would enhance my understanding of patients and my approach to their care. Perhaps the greatest contribution that acupuncture can make to Western medicine is not simply the addition of another useful new technique, but an expansion of how we perceive the nature and functioning of the body.

10

Man's Natural Diet

Man's Natural Diet

Diet is an essential influence on our health, so what foods should we eat? What is the ideal diet for a human being? The answer is not immediately obvious. In any bookstore today, you are likely to find shelves of books on the subject of nutrition, each with a somewhat different opinion on how people should eat. Every authority seems to have his own ideas on the subject, and it is confusing to decide whom to believe.

Such disagreement is possible because human beings can eat so many different kinds of food. This capacity distinguishes us from most other animals. A deer eats grass or other plants, a tiger eats meat, and a bird eats seeds and fruit, and none of them could exchange diets with any other. But a human being may eat and survive on all of these foods.

Because we are capable of digesting and utilizing such a variety of foods, it is possible to consider any of them as a natural food for us. However, though they may all support life, their effects upon the body will not be the same. We can survive on many kinds of food, but the quality of our existence will be influenced considerably by which ones we choose. Some diet must be the most "natural" for people to eat, in the sense that it allows the highest level of physical and emotional health.

For animals, determining a natural diet is easy. They seem to know intuitively what they should eat. Unlike human beings, they do not need a book on nutrition for advice on their diet. Presumably, our distant ancestors once possessed such instincts, but human beings today, and especially those of us in a modern society, have lost most of this ability. We have replaced intuition with reason, and must now rely upon our intellectual capacities to tell us how to eat.

One way to find clues to a good diet is to examine how people before us have eaten. The diet of our earliest ancestors was probably a lot like that of our nearest biological relatives, the great apes: a broadly omnivorous diet consisting of fruits, nuts, wild plants, insects, and perhaps occasional meat.

In one sense, this could be considered our most "natural" diet. But it is only possible in parts of the world with a relatively tropical climate. As early humans moved into colder climates, this diet was no longer available, and it was also less appropriate for a colder environment. People were obliged to turn to hunting and eating other animals that were better adapted for survival in these colder surroundings.

Eventually early hunting societies began to domesticate wild plants and grow their own food. This marked another major change in how people ate. With the appearance of agriculture, people developed diets that utilized the plants that grew easily where they lived. While these diets varied widely in different parts of the world, it is interesting that most of them shared certain essential features. In nearly all agricultural societies, the cereal grasses, in one form or another, assumed a primary role. Thus, for thousands of years, human beings almost everywhere have relied upon various grains as their staple food.

Rice has traditionally been the basic food for the people of China and East Asia, while corn was the primary food grown in the Americas. Wheat and rye were used widely in Europe and the Middle East, and various other grains, including barley, oats, millet, and buckwheat, have also been staple foods in different parts of the world. Even today, grains make up a large part of the diet for most of the world, although they are conspicuously absent from the modern American diet. In Japan the symbol for a "meal" is identical with that for "rice," indicating that originally the concept of a meal was synonymous with eating rice. And in the West the Bible describes bread, which is made from grain, as the "staff of life."

Another food traditionally grown throughout the world is legumes (beans, peas, lentils, etc.). We now know that grains and legumes eaten together are a particularly good combination. When these two food groups are combined, they provide an excellent source of complete protein that is otherwise lacking in vegetable foods, because each of them supplies amino acids that are absent in the other. This property of protein complementarity is a recent discovery of biochemistry and one in which modern vegetarians have become especially interested.

But for thousands of years before this, people around the world have recognized the value of this combination, and have relied upon these foods as the foundation of their diet. In Mexico and much of South America, one finds a traditional diet based upon the combination of corn (a grain) and beans (a legume), and in India people rely extensively on meals of rice (grain) and lentils (legume). This pattern occurs repeatedly in the diets of many other traditional cultures.

In addition to grains and legumes, people have eaten fruits and vegetables, first as wild plants and later by cultivating their own crops. Depending upon geography, they may also have eaten fish, as well as some meat. As some traditional cultures began to keep domestic animals for the purpose of giving milk, dairy products were also introduced to the diet in certain areas.

Despite regional differences, the fundamental structure of most traditional diets is quite similar. Whole grains, legumes, and other vegetable foods are eaten in large amounts, while animal foods, such as meat and dairy products, make up a relatively small part of the diet. Meals consist almost entirely of foods that can be found locally, and they are generally eaten in the seasons when they are naturally available. Processed foods such as white flour, refined sugar, or synthetic food additives do not play any part in the diet, and until recently were unknown in the diets of people anywhere. Even in America, artificial food additives were rarely used until the beginning of this century, and did not come into widespread use until after World War II.

This is obviously very different from what we consider a normal diet today. Taking a long-range perspective on history, we can see our modern diet as a sort of nutritional aberration—an abrupt departure from the diet eaten by people for thousands of years before us. We can also see that today's so-called "health food" diets are not really anything new, but simply attempts to return to what has always been a traditional human diet.

It is ironic that while these foods are often portrayed as passing health "fads," they have far more historical basis than the diet we accept as normal. In terms of human history, the true "fad diet" is actually the one most often consumed today.

Much of the change in our diet has resulted from changes in how we get our food. Food production has passed from the hands of individual families to become a form of big business, often carried on by large corporations. It involves a complex system of growing, distributing, and marketing products across the world. Often, the food we eat may have been grown hundreds or even thousands of miles away.

These changes have meant that most food now goes through a great deal of processing and packaging before it reaches the person who actually eats it, and it is rarely eaten in its natural state. Mass-produced foods—soft drinks, instant mixes, packaged breakfast cereals, and many other products that until recently did not even exist —have become common items in our diet.

In the past, diets were simpler. The enormous variety of products we now take for granted in any supermarket was not available. Of necessity, people were closer to the source of what they ate, and there was no time gap between production and consumption of food. The idea of food as something that comes in a box or a can on the supermarket shelf would have been incomprehensible to our ancestors. By being directly involved with obtaining their own food, they could recognize that what they ate were parts of living plants or animals to which human beings had a biological connection.

Today we are more confused about what food is. But while we may no longer have an intuitive sense of what to eat, we do know a great deal about the biochemistry of nutrition. We can use this knowledge to understand why our ancestors maintained certain principles in their diet, and how these same principles can be restored to our present way of eating.

Optimal Nutrition

The three classes of nutrients in any food are proteins, fats, and carbohydrates. In a traditional diet based primarily on whole grains, legumes, and vegetables, the major ingredients are starches and other complex carbohydrates. Simple carbohydrates, or sugars, are present, but to a lesser extent. The diet also contains protein and fats, but these are included in relatively small amounts as compared to carbohydrates. Because the diet consists chiefly of fresh foods, it is likely to provide abundant vitamins and minerals, as well as large amounts of fiber.

In terms of what we know of biochemistry, this diet seems well suited to our nutritional needs. These needs fall into two general categories: food as a source of energy, and food to maintain our bodies. The bulk of what we eat is utilized to fuel the body's life processes. Carbohydrates are the most accessible form of this energy, and anything else must first be converted by the body to this form.

Thus carbohydrates represent the most appropriate food to eat for energy. They are also the "cleanest" metabolically, in terms of producing the fewest waste products to be eliminated when they are burned by the body. Because most of what we eat is used this way, it seems reasonable that a large proportion of our diet should be complex carbohydrates.

Fats and protein can also be used for energy, but they are actually required for a different purpose. This is the second function of food—to meet the structural needs of the body. Many tissues of the body are made of fats and proteins, and these are needed to replace cellular structures as they are broken down.

The requirements for fats and protein, as well as for micronutrients such as vitamins and minerals, are quite specific. However, they are relatively small compared to the quantity of food needed for energy. While it is essential to have enough fats and protein, it is also desirable to avoid too much. An optimal balance of nutrients would include large amounts of complex carbohydrates for energy, with enough fats and protein to meet the body's structural requirements, but not so much as to create an excess. It would also include necessary vitamins and minerals, as well as plenty of fiber.

A traditional human diet provides this balance of nutrients, but even a casual look at our modern diet shows how these proportions have been drastically altered and even reversed. Rather than grains and vegetables, our diet is centered upon meat and dairy products, which provide a much higher proportion of protein and fats. In addition, concentrated fats such as butter, oils, margarine, or mayonnaise are widely used. And naturally occurring complex carbohydrates have been replaced by refined sugar.

A typical dinner today might consist of steak, fried potatoes, a bit of cooked vegetable, white bread and butter, cake for dessert, and coffee sweetened with sugar. Though each of these foods may not necessarily be unhealthy, the overall effect of this meal is a most inappropriate balance of nutrients. It is high in fat, high in protein, and high in sugar; it contains few complex carbohydrates; and it is likely to be deficient in fiber and in various vitamins and minerals. If this kind of meal is eaten consistently, it is inevitable that an imbalance will exist in the diet.

To correct this, it is necessary to look at the diet as a whole. I am often asked whether this or that food is "good" to eat, but these questions only make sense in the context of the entire diet. It can be misleading to concentrate only on specific foods.

The controversy over heart disease and fats in the diet is an excellent example. When this association began to receive publicity, many people became sufficiently alarmed to make changes in their diet. Butter was named as a particular culprit, and millions of families switched to margarine, which was promoted as a healthy alternative. The idea that butter is bad and margarine is good became popularly accepted.

Now it seems this was too simple. Margarine is made by artificially saturating vegetable oils, so that they will become solid at room temperature, and appear similar to butter. However, this process produces a substance with a molecular structure that does not normally exist in nature, and its effect on human biochemistry is not entirely understood. There is now a question whether the synthetic fats in margarine may contribute even more to the development of heart disease than those in butter. And as research continues, the conclusions about which fats are more harmful than others will probably change from year to year.

But all of this misses the main point. It is not a question of whether butter or margarine is intrinsically good or bad. It is that when one abandons a natural diet, one of the many consequences of the resulting imbalance can be the development of heart disease. This will not be prevented by substituting a stick of margarine for a stick of butter. It can only be accomplished by restructuring the composition of the diet as a whole.

The Foundation of Our Meals

People often try to change their diet by singling out specific foods. While one decides to give up butter, another will avoid sugar, and still another will eat less red meat. Each of these changes may be helpful, but they are still a fragmented approach to diet. We eliminate one food after another because it is "bad," but still do not understand what to eat in its place.

The lack of a solid dietary foundation is especially apparent in the remarkable absence of whole grains from our diet. The food that has for thousands of years provided the nutritional basis for human societies is almost totally missing from our meals. For most people today, the only significant source of grains is white bread and packaged breakfast cereals. However, these are both highly processed, devitalized foods that have lost most of their nutritional value.

As my own understanding of nutrition has evolved, one of the most profound changes in my diet has been the rediscovery of whole grains. These now provide a solid center for my meals, to which all other foods may be added, and I have learned to recognize them as the most basic of human foods. I relish a steaming bowl of cooked grains in the morning. Their solidity and chewy sweetness seem to convey the essential flavors and textures of the earth. Eating this food, I feel in touch with how my ancestors and those of all human beings have eaten.

It is sad that instead of such food, the people of America have somehow come to accept that breakfast consists of dry, processed, sugared flakes packaged in a brightly colored box. Although we refer to this food as "cereal," it is far from the original meaning of the word, which refers to plants that bear the seeds that provide our whole grains. These hardy plants grow everywhere across the world, and in any vacant lot you can find the wild grasses that are the distant ancestors of wheat, rye, and other grains we now know. Through thousands of years of selection, these grasses were cultivated into the food plants familiar to so many generations of human beings.

Perhaps more than anything in a meal, different grains somehow capture the essence of the cultures they have nourished. Eating a bowl of buckwheat and whole wheat noodles, for example, I imagine my own great-grandparents and the generations before them sustained by a dish identical to this through the cold winters of Eastern Europe. Other cultures have chosen different grains as the foundation of their diet, by domesticating the local plants that were available to them.

In traditional cultures, grains were not simply the foods people happened to eat in large quantity. They held a role of unique importance, and were credited with special symbolic and spiritual significance in the lives and rituals of the people. Other foods might or might not be available, but grains invariably provided the basis of any meal.

According to Oriental medicine, whole grains are the most inherently balanced of all foods; thus, they are singularly appropriate to serve as the foundation of the diet. And from the standpoint of Western nutrition, they contain an optimal combination of nutrients. Each kernel of rice, wheat, or corn is a seed from which an entire new plant could grow, and its construction reflects this purpose. At the heart of each seed is the "germ" (as in "wheat germ"), which contains the genetic material for the entire plant. It is a highly concentrated source of protein, oils, and various vitamins, and although quite small, it contains a large portion of the nutrients present in the grain.

Surrounding the germ is a bulky mass of starches and other complex carbohydrates. This serves as a source of energy for the growing sprout, until it is large enough to put out leaves and draw its energy from the sun. The final component of each grain is a tough, protective outer layer referred to as the "bran." This outer coating contains various vitamins as well as large amounts of fiber.

Thus each grain contains the same overall balance we want in our total diet—much complex carbohydrate for energy, plenty of fiber, small amounts of protein and fat, and a good supply of various vitamins and minerals. While it would be too limited to live entirely on grains, it is apparent that they can make up a large part of the diet.

Unfortunately, most grains eaten today go through processing that destroys this excellent balance. Grains are usually turned into flour, which typically involves removing the germ and the bran, and then grinding the remainder. Along the way, they may also be treated with preservatives and other additives. The product that results can sit on the shelf for a long time without spoiling, but it has lost most of the nutrients found in the marvelously balanced whole grain.

The absence of grains in our diet is not the only departure from the past. Our unique blend of cuisines derived from a variety of cultural traditions has been overwhelmed by an onslaught of mass-produced, processed foods and "fast foods," which are now the closest thing we have to a national diet. This has not only made our diet less interesting, but has had serious consequences for our health, as seen in the epidemic of degenerative diseases we are now experiencing.

The response of our health care system to this problem has been limited, and nutrition remains a neglected area in medical education. I learned about specific deficiency diseases in medical school, but the broader and more fundamental question of what constitutes a healthy diet for human beings was not addressed. Nutritional education was based on the vague assumption that any reasonably varied diet that met minimal requirements was adequate, and that no further attention to nutrition was needed beyond this.

In the past, there was perhaps some basis for such an assumption. Most food was eaten in a relatively natural state, and you did not have to go to a special store to buy "health food" or "natural food." You could not live on candy bars and soft drinks and TV dinners, as people can today, because these foods did not exist. The main concern in regard to food was simply getting enough of it.

So it is not surprising that in the past, medicine has focused on diseases involving deficiencies in the diet. However, today it is easy for people in this country not only to get enough to eat, but to eat far more than they need, especially foods that are inappropriate for good nutrition. Thus, we are discovering new medical problems caused not only by deficiencies but by excess. People are eating too much sugar, too much fat, too much meat, too much salt, too much processed food, and perhaps simply too much food of all kinds.

Helping people to arrive at a balance between excess and deficiency in their diet is an important part of medical care. Sound nutritional advice should be far more sophisticated than a simple description of the four food groups, but unfortunately doctors usually pay little attention to what their patients are eating. Thus, people must learn for themselves what constitutes a healthy way to eat, and which foods are best to choose for their personal diet.

Choosing a Personal Diet

Proper nutrition provides a foundation for good health. While a nutritious diet alone may not guarantee health, it at least creates the conditions in which health can exist. Similarly, poor diet will make it difficult, if not impossible, for anyone to maintain good health indefinitely.

I am continually reminded of this in my medical practice. I ask all new patients to complete a questionnaire about their medical history, which includes several questions about diet. But I rarely need to look at the answers to learn how they eat. The answer is evident not only in the presence of certain medical problems, but in the texture of the skin, the sparkle of the eyes, the tone of the muscles, and a hundred other subtle and not so subtle clues that reveal the story of the body's health to the careful observer. This is particularly true for older people, whose faces and bodies reflect the accumulated effects of how they have lived for many years.

These effects are dramatic. The differences between those who have eaten well and those who have not can be enormous. I am repeatedly impressed by the ravages of improper diet. I am also impressed by what can be accomplished through changes in diet. People willing to change to a more natural way of eating can be helped significantly with many specific medical problems. Invariably, they will also feel better. After improving their diet, many people feel lighter and have more energy. They also may be more relaxed, or sleep better, or move their bowels more easily, or notice a host of other improvements.

Beginning these changes is usually the most difficult part of creating a better diet. Habits can become firmly established, and many people have fallen into an unhealthy pattern of eating that is far removed from a natural diet. Major changes may be needed in their choice of food and even in their concept of what constitutes a meal. For the person who thinks of food in terms of fast-food hamburgers, soft drinks, and candy bars, it is a great leap to consider eating whole grains, legumes, and vegetables instead. For most people, changes of this magnitude cannot realistically be accomplished at once, but must be approached in gradual steps. This allows the changes to become part of the daily routine on a more permanent basis.

The precise make-up of an optimal diet varies somewhat from one individual to another, and no single diet fits everyone. Nutritional needs depend upon age, sex, physical activity, and body type. They also will change for the same person in different environmental conditions and with the seasons of the year. However, the basic outline of an appropriate diet for human beings remains essentially the same for us all. The following recommendations can be helpful for anyone in their choice of food:

1. Eat foods as close to their natural state as possible. Avoid products that have been highly processed or refined, and instead eat more whole foods that retain their natural balance of nutrients. Whole wheat, for example, is a whole food, as opposed to white flour, which is a refined product made from the whole food, and contains only a fraction of its original nutrients.

2. Base your diet upon simple foods, including whole grains, vegetables, beans, and fruits. Foods eaten in addition to these basic foods should be used in comparatively small amounts.

3. Milk products, including milk, cheese, or yogurt, are not well tolerated by some people who have difficulty digesting them properly. If you have no problem with them, they are a good source of protein and other nutrients. However, they are very concentrated foods that are quite high in fat. Because they are convenient to eat, it is easy to consume far too many dairy products, so they are best eaten only in moderation.

4. It is also best to eat meat in small amounts, rather than as the center of your meals. Fish and poultry are a better choice than red meat, which is much higher in fat.

If you prefer not to eat meat, an intelligently planned vegetarian diet is one of the healthiest ways you can eat. However, if you do not eat meat, you should be sure that your diet contains a proper balance of protein from other sources to meet your needs.

5. Avoid highly processed foods such as sugar, white flour products, convenience foods, or "junk food" snacks. Generally try to minimize the amount of canned, packaged, or prepared foods in your diet, especially those containing preservatives and artificial additives.

6. Eat primarily the foods that can grow in the climate where you live. In addition, change your diet somewhat with the seasons, so that your meals are appropriate to the time of year. Raw fruits and vegetables, juices, or salads are normally available in the summer, and are good food for hot weather. They are less appropriate as a regular diet in the winter months, when we need more substantial meals. Foods like dried beans and grains, potatoes, and other root vegetables are normally available during the winter, and should be eaten more during cold weather.

7. Maintain a balance in your diet so that you will get enough of all necessary nutrients, but not too much of anything. Eating too much of certain foods, such as fats or refined sugar, can place a strain on the body's digestion and metabolism and can lead to problems of overweight and illness.

These are general guidelines for eating that can be modified to meet your own personal needs and preferences. They should not be looked at as strict rules, but as a basic foundation for choosing a diet that will be healthy and satisfying.

Healing with Food

Doctors could provide most help to their patients in the area of nutrition by educating them in the principles of a natural human diet. However, most diets prescribed by doctors are designed to relieve symptoms, rather than improve the patient's health through better nutrition.

In medical school I learned about specific diets for people with certain kinds of illness. Now many of these diets, which have long been a part of medical practice, are being seriously questioned. Perhaps the classic example is the well-known bland diet for peptic ulcers, in which the patient eats large amounts of milk and dairy products, while many other foods are eliminated.

For years, this diet was the foundation of ulcer treatment and was routinely prescribed for millions of people. When I was a student, it would have been unthinkable to question its value. But a remarkable reversal has taken place. It has now been concluded that the bland diet does not benefit people with ulcers and its use is no longer recommended. It is even thought to create an increased risk of heart disease or other problems because of its high fat content.

Having been unequivocally taught that a bland diet was necessary for people with ulcers, I find this reversal in thinking particularly instructive. It is a good reminder of how thoroughly medical theories can change. Only a few years ago, anyone who seriously questioned the usefulness of a bland diet would have been met with derision. Yet anyone who still prescribes this diet now may experience the same disapproval.

What is accepted without question one day may be discarded a few years later, and it is likely that many of today's firmly held beliefs in medicine will meet this same fate at some time in the future. It is valuable to keep the transitory nature of medical theories in mind. It helps to maintain an open mind toward new ideas and a willingness to question the beliefs of the day.

Another diet that has also recently been abandoned is the low-residue diet for people with diverticulitis. This is a common condition in which small pouches, known as diverticuli, form in the lining of the large intestine. These pouches may become infected, causing pain and occasionally more serious complications. As a student, I was taught that people with diverticulitis should be put on a diet low in residue, or fiber. The idea was that particles of fiber might become trapped in the diverticuli and produce inflammation. People were advised to stick to soft foods, and avoid such things as whole grains, raw fruits and vegetables, and nuts or seeds.

At the time, this theory appeared to make sense, but we now know that this is precisely the type of diet that *causes* diverticulitis. In cultures that eat unprocessed foods high in fiber, diverticulitis is one of the many intestinal diseases that does not occur. Thus, we were instructing people to exaggerate the very diet that had caused the problem in the first place. Now we realize that a *high-residue* diet is needed to maintain proper intestinal function. Thus most people with diverticulitis are encouraged to do the opposite of what they used to be told and include abundant fiber in their diet.

Still another example of how dietary theories can change is seen in the treatment of diabetes. At one time, people with diabetes were told to avoid eating carbohydrates, but otherwise they could pretty much do as they pleased with their diet. Because the most obvious sign of diabetes is elevated blood sugar, this seemed to make sense. However, it failed to make the crucial distinction between carbohydrate in the form of refined sugar and the naturally occurring complex carbohydrates. It is now apparent that while diabetics should avoid sugar, complex carbohydrates in the form of grains, vegetables, or other foods may have a beneficial effect and help to stabilize blood sugar.

Diabetes turns out to be more complex than was once thought, affecting many aspects of the body's biochemistry. Metabolism of fats is also involved, so that not only is it necessary to avoid sugar, but a low-fat diet also seems helpful.

The old recommendation to diabetics to stay away from carbohydrates, but eat whatever else they wanted, was not only too simple, but actually incorrect and probably even harmful. It may be that for years we were telling people with diabetes to eat the wrong foods, while avoiding the foods that would be most helpful for them.

The different diets described here follow the same pattern. They are all examples of widely prescribed diets that have proved ineffective in accomplishing their purpose. For some people, they may even have contributed to worsening their illness. All have been unsuccessful because they are based upon a limited perspective. They are designed to counteract certain obvious symptoms of disease, rather than influence the overall functioning of the whole person.

A more effective approach would be to prescribe a diet to improve the total health of the patient. This does not mean one diet is prescribed for people with peptic ulcer, another for diverticulitis, and still another for diabetes. Instead the diet that seems most helpful for each of these, and for many other medical conditions as well, turns out to be very much the same. This is nothing more than the traditional diet human beings have consumed throughout history, which has only recently been lost to us in the modern world.

This is an enormously important conclusion. It means that with certain exceptions, there really are not specific diets for specific diseases. The same diet that leads to optimal functioning of all aspects of the body will be helpful in treating most any disease.

In a sense, it is almost too simple. People continue to look for a special new diet, or a different vitamin supplement, or a detailed biochemical analysis of their nutritional state. While these all may be appropriate in some situations, they are not the answer to achieving optimal nutrition and health for most of us. This will only be achieved by returning to the simple, natural diet that has sustained countless generations of human beings before us.

11

Protecting Your
Personal Health

Practicing True Preventive Medicine

As a doctor, a part of my job is to help people understand
how they can prevent different diseases. This is an essential part of health care, as it is always much easier to
prevent a problem than it is to take care of it once it exists.
It is also important to realize the extent to which our most
serious diseases can be prevented.

In a previous chapter, we examined the possible risk
factors for coronary artery disease, the single leading
cause of death in America. These included cigarette
smoking, lack of physical exercise, overweight, a high-fat
diet, and chronic emotional stress. All of these are potentially within the control of any individual. Thus, while
heart disease remains statistically a major cause of death,
it is possible for an individual person to adopt a lifestyle
that will make this disease perhaps not impossible, but at
least unlikely.

The same is true of other serious forms of cardio-
vascular disease. Many of the risk factors for strokes or
for circulatory problems in the legs are the same as those
for coronary artery disease, and the same changes that

can prevent heart disease can help prevent these as well. Millions of Americans end their lives crippled by strokes that could have been prevented. Probably the single greatest cause of these strokes is cigarette smoking. The rate of strokes among smokers is far higher than among nonsmokers, and even if no other changes are made, simply stopping smoking can greatly reduce the likelihood of an eventual stroke. This can be helpful even if one has already been a smoker for a long period of time. If changes are also made in other risk factors, the possibility of a stroke, like that of heart disease, becomes increasingly unlikely.

Our awareness of the value of preventive medicine is steadily increasing and we seem to be hearing more about it all the time. However, a great deal of what is presented as preventive medicine today is misnamed. It does not really have anything to do with *prevention* of illness, but rather with its *early detection*.

Getting a yearly chest X-ray, for example, may allow early detection of lung cancer, but it does not do anything to prevent the disease. To quit smoking cigarettes, on the other hand, is a form of actual prevention. Similarly, regular sigmoidoscope exams are a means of early detection of intestinal cancer. Eating a high-fiber, low-fat diet is a means of prevention. Examining your own breasts and getting periodic mammograms (breast X-rays) can help in early detection of breast cancer. A low-fat diet as well as breast feeding your children can be effective forms of prevention.

Various tests for early diagnosis of cancer, as well as other diseases, are certainly valuable. The earlier a problem is discovered, the more likely it is to be treated successfully. But these tests are not preventive medicine. They do nothing to actually prevent the appearance of disease; they only diagnose it sooner when it does appear. True preventive medicine can only be practiced by the patient himself. It has little to do with doctors, although the doctor can certainly help in explaining what must be done, but it does relate to the quality of life.

Understanding the Risk Factors for Cancer

Perhaps we are more conscious today of the prevalence of cancer than any other disease. The factors involved in developing cancer are complex and not entirely understood, but we know enough to recognize that it is a good deal more preventable than many people may realize. Among American men, the most common form of cancer involves the lung, and the association of lung cancer with smoking cigarettes has become common knowledge. Although it does occur among nonsmokers, lung cancer is relatively unusual in this group.

Lung cancer is also associated with chronic exposure to certain substances in the air. Asbestos particles are a well-known and particularly notorious example, and many people today suffer from lung cancer or other lung diseases caused by exposure to asbestos at work. Simultaneous exposure to more than one carcinogen can have a particularly devastating effect. Cigarette smokers who have also been exposed to asbestos or other industrial carcinogens develop lung cancer with much greater frequency than those exposed to only one of these factors. Most people with lung cancer either have been smokers or have a history of exposure to carcinogens in the air, typically at their place of work. Thus it seems clear what must be done to avoid this disease. On a statistical basis, a person who does not smoke and does not work in an environment with toxic chemicals in the air is unlikely to develop lung cancer.

The situation is similar for various other cancers of the head, neck, and throat. Many of these are also associated with smoking, excessive use of alcohol, and especially with both at the same time. These are particularly unpleasant diseases, but to a considerable extent they are also preventable. For the person who does not smoke and does not drink to excess, they are another disease that is relatively unlikely to appear.

Smoking can also contribute to cancers in more remote parts of the body. Bladder cancer, for example, seems to have a higher incidence among smokers, and may also develop after exposure to certain toxic substances. Once again, an understanding of the causes allows us to see what must be done to prevent the disease, or at least make it less likely.

In an earlier chapter we saw that cancer of the colon is extremely rare in cultures that follow a certain diet and lifestyle. The typical modern diet that is high in fats, sugar, and processed foods, while lacking fiber and unrefined food, appears to be the chief culprit. Epidemiological evidence suggests that a change to a more natural diet could make this disease as rare in America as it is in other parts of the world. Thus, through attention to proper diet, any individual can help protect himself against what is today the most common form of cancer in this country.

Evidence suggests that our modern diet predisposes us to other forms of cancer as well. Breast cancer, for example, has in the past been largely attributed to hereditary or hormonal factors. While these play an important part, it appears that another factor in the appearance of breast cancer is diet. A high-fat diet has been particularly implicated, although most women remain unaware of this connection.

Whether or not a woman breastfeeds her children may also be a factor in the development of breast cancer. Women who do not have children or who do not breastfeed appear to have a statistically higher incidence of breast cancer than those who do. Somehow this lack of use of the breast for its natural function may create a situation that predisposes to disease. So among the benefits of breastfeeding for both mother and child, we can also include at least some degree of protection against cancer.

The list of preventable cancers could go on at length. There is, for example, an association between skin cancer and prolonged exposure to ultraviolet light. It is especially important for people with fair complexions to avoid excessive exposure to the sun in order to decrease the possibility of this disease. Cancer of the liver is commonly seen in people who drink too much alcohol or have been exposed to various carcinogens. Cancer of the pancreas has a higher incidence among heavy smokers. Again, understanding the risk factors tells us what must be done to avoid the diseases.

Another contributing factor for some cases of cancer is radiation. Exposure to radiation, whether in the form of medical X-rays, at work, or perhaps even in the home, can lead to the eventual appearance of cancer. Thyroid cancer, for example, can often be traced to radiation to the neck years earlier. This procedure was once performed commonly as a treatment for such conditions as enlarged tonsils and adenoids, acne, or fungus infections, before its risks were understood.

Exposure to radiation can occur in strange and unexpected ways. In the past, watches and clocks with luminous dials were made with radium, which glows in the dark. The radium was applied to the hands of the clock in the form of a paint, and the workers who painted the clocks would lick the tip of their brush to bring it to a fine point. Over the years, many of them gradually ingested significant amounts of radioactive radium and eventually developed various forms of cancer as a result.

Because most radiation is received today in the form of medical X-rays, the obvious place to begin avoiding it is by not having unnecessary X-rays. However, this is not always easy. When a patient arrives at his office, one of the first things a doctor, dentist, or chiropractor will often do is order X-rays. Sometimes this is necessary. In some situations X-rays are extremely useful for diagnosing a problem, and nothing else can provide the same information. But a great many X-rays are ordered as a matter of convenience or routine, and could be avoided with some thought on the part of the doctor or dentist.

Until recently, for example, any patient admitted to a hospital for any reason automatically had a chest X-ray. This added up to an enormous number of chest X-rays. Now we are realizing that not only is this not necessary, but the cumulative effects of such routine radiation may be dangerous.

While chest X-rays involve a relatively small amount of radiation, there are other, more elaborate X-rays that require far higher levels of exposure. If you visit the doctor complaining of digestive problems, one of the first things he may do is order an upper GI study, a series of X-rays that view the stomach and intestines from various directions and involve significant radiation. While these are sometimes necessary, they are often ordered without consideration for the fact that they involve a certain hazard for the patient. It is an unfortunate tendency to order the X-rays first and then think about the problem, rather than the other way around.

Because of this, the patient may need to take an active role in protecting himself, and make it clear that he does not want X-rays unless they are absolutely necessary. This may require asking questions when X-rays are ordered. It is important to be sure that your doctor is X-raying your sprained ankle because he really thinks it may be broken, and not because he routinely does this for any sprained ankle. And it is important to let your dentist know that you do not want X-rays every time you sit down in his chair, but only if there is some specific problem that legitimately requires an X-ray for diagnosis. The same applies to a chiropractor. These small steps could conceivably help prevent serious disease years later.

Whatever the contributing factor may be, a certain

pattern appears throughout this discussion of how different cancers might be prevented. When we develop cancer, it is often because in some way our bodies have not been treated properly. We are exposed to radiation or smoke cigarettes or drink too much alcohol or eat the wrong diet or come in contact with harmful chemicals in the air or water. If we take all the different cancers for which such causes are clearly identified, it becomes apparent that at least a substantial percentage of them can be prevented by our individual actions.

It is estimated that approximately one in four Americans today will develop cancer. This is a very frightening statistic, but the rate need not be nearly that high if we lived in a healthier manner. Many millions of dollars are spent every year to fund a small army of researchers who investigate cures for cancer, but the means of prevention are already at hand if we would only pay attention to them. If you eat a healthy, natural diet, do not smoke, do not drink alcohol to excess, and avoid exposure to radiation or dangerous chemicals, you will, with these simple measures, dramatically decrease the likelihood of developing the most common cancers in our society.

Taking Responsibility for Your Health

The same measures that may prevent cancer can also help prevent most of the other leading causes of illness and death today. Heart disease, strokes, diabetes, ulcers, intestinal disease, chronic lung disease, gall bladder or liver disease—practically any of our major diseases can be related to factors of diet, lifestyle, environment, and emotional state.

To a surprising degree, this is even true of accidents or injuries. While working as an Emergency Room physician, I inevitably saw many people who had had accidents of some kind. Anyone who spends much time at this work soon realizes that these accidents do not just happen with no reason. Most of the time people are injured in certain situations—typically when their behavior has been influenced by alcohol or drugs, or by some strong emotion. They usually find themselves in the Emergency Room when they are drunk, angry, or upset, or when they have had the misfortune to encounter someone else in such a state.

Several years ago I broke a toe. As I was preparing for bed one evening, I felt angry about an incident earlier in the day and strode across the room, preoccupied with my thoughts. With my attention elsewhere, my bare foot slammed into the bedpost, breaking the little toe. It was an abrupt and painful reminder to wake up and pay attention. Although my broken toe was an "accident," it clearly would not have happened had I been in a different emotional state.

Many accidents can be viewed in this way. If you are fortunate enough to have only a small accident, you can take it as a warning to pay attention, and hopefully avoid another reminder that may be more serious. Accidents, like illnesses, can sometimes be prevented. This prevention often involves the same habits and emotional attitudes that help to keep you healthy in other ways.

Childbirth and Preventive Medicine

It is never too early in life to begin paying attention to the prevention of medical problems. Indeed, it should logically begin with pregnancy and childbirth. Reproduction is a biological function, like digestion or breathing. If our bodies are cared for properly, then all organ systems, including those of reproduction, will work at their best. A woman who has cared for herself well through pregnancy, and who enters labor in good health, will be far less likely to suffer complications.

What distinguishes childbirth from other normal biological activities is that it involves a relatively short period of intense physical and psychological exertion. Therefore it requires special preparation. In many parts of the world, women's bodies are already prepared for this exertion by the physical demands of their daily existence, and they are prepared mentally by living in cultures where the birth process is a familiar event. In America we have a more sedentary lifestyle, and childbirth is hidden away in the confines of hospitals. Thus, special preparation involving education, diet, and exercise may be necessary.

Like most medical problems, those associated with pregnancy or childbirth are often the result of the individual's lifestyle. Everything the mother eats, drinks, or experiences during her pregnancy will also reach the baby in her womb and affect it in some way. And in its vulnerable condition of development, the baby may be susceptible to influences that the mature body of the mother has learned to tolerate.

The pregnant mother must pay unusually careful attention to good diet and regular physical exercise, and she must eliminate the use of potentially harmful drugs, including alcohol, tobacco, and caffeine. She should also try to avoid situations likely to provoke strong negative emotions. Many traditional cultures have long accepted the idea that emotions, like food, can be transmitted from the mother to the baby inside her. If one accepts this premise, then it seems as inappropriate to see a pregnant woman in a theater watching a particularly violent or gruesome movie as it does to see her smoking a cigarette. As in so many other areas of life, avoiding behaviors that compromise personal health and predispose one to illness is the secret to prevention of medical problems further down the line.

The Quality of Life

There is, of course, no guarantee that anything you do will lead to good health or a long life. Despite the most careful pregnancy, a person may be born with some congenital abnormality. Or you may get in the way of someone else's negative emotions and be struck down in an accident. And no matter how much you try to follow a healthy lifestyle, you may still get sick. Lean, muscular long-distance runners have collapsed from a heart attack, and health food enthusiasts who watch their diet for years have died of cancer.

No single factor is *the* answer to maintaining health. There is more to it than diet alone, or exercise alone, or any other single consideration. Good health and longevity result from the complex interaction of many factors, including some that we may never be able to completely understand or control.

But though there are no guarantees for any individual, we can, at least on a statistical basis, make certain choices that will increase our chances for a long and healthy life. These choices will influence not only life expectancy, but also the quality of our life. We must all die in the end, so our concern is not only for how many years we will live but what those years will be like. The robust old man on the bicycle described at the beginning of this book was remarkable not for his age, but for what he was still able to do at that age. He had remained vigorous and fully immersed in life to an extent most people would find extraordinary. Yet what he was doing is potentially within the reach of many others.

Theories about the aging process and how to counteract it seem particularly popular these days. However, I must confess to a certain skepticism about some of the ideas being proposed. Some programs claim to maintain health and prevent aging through an enormous variety of nutritional supplements and synthetic chemicals. Although only time will tell whether such an approach has merit, my guess is that it is not the answer for most of us.

Actually the secret of longevity may really be no secret, but a way of living that some people have understood and successfully followed throughout history. It is simpler than any elaborate program of supplements, but also much more difficult to accomplish. To lead a long and healthy life, one must provide the body with an appropriate diet for its daily functioning—not too much, not too little, and composed of a good balance of simple foods in their natural state. One must also use the body as it was meant to be used. This means physical exercise that affects all parts of the body: exercises that keep the muscles strong and flexible, while stimulating nerves, blood vessels, and glands; exercises that move the breath freely and deeply through the lungs. It also means avoiding regular use of harmful substances, such as drugs, excessive alcohol, tobacco, toxic chemicals, or unhealthy foods. Finally, one must maintain a healthy emotional equilibrium and avoid becoming caught up too often in anger, fear, depression, or other negative internal states.

This last is perhaps the most difficult for most of us. We assume that our emotional states are an automatic reaction to external events and, as such, are largely outside our control. However, this is not entirely true. Just as we influence our internal *physical* environment through the food we eat and the care we give our body, we can also learn in more subtle ways to influence the internal *emotional* environment.

Maintaining a Balance

Longevity requires a state in which the body is in physical and emotional balance. Various methods exist that encourage such a balance. Appropriate diet is obviously one of these, and this has already been discussed in some detail. In addition, many specific physical activities will promote good health. Various forms of meditation or spiritual practice can also help maintain this balance.

Recently, interest in physical exercise has increased dramatically in America, and everywhere you see people running, bicycling, swimming, or attending exercise classes. This has had an extremely positive effect upon our collective health. The benfits of regular vigorous exercise, both for physical fitness and emotional well-being, are enormous. For many people, this has become an important way to take responsibility for their own health.

Various practices from Eastern cultures have also been introduced in America, and have become increasingly popular. The physical postures and breathing exercises of hatha yoga, or the Taoist exercises and martial arts of China such as t'ai chi ch'uan, not only build strength and endurance, but are said to stimulate movement of the life force, the *prana* or *chi*, throughout the body. These practices represent a highly effective form of preventive medicine.

The postures of hatha yoga stimulate the breath, the blood flow, and the nervous system, stretch each muscle and joint of the body, straighten the spine, and massage and invigorate the various internal organs and glands. What more could one ask of a system of exercise as a health practice? Although yoga or t'ai chi ch'uan are not taught in Western medical schools, I find them increasingly relevant to the practice of medicine. They are an approach to health and longevity that has been proven over many centuries.

As a physician, I may help a patient to correct some symptom of illness through my treatment. But if the underlying condition of the body remains the same, it may eventually express itself in other forms of illness. In order to encourage more permanent change in the body I will sometimes introduce patients to selected exercises, perhaps chosen from hatha yoga. Such exercises can be very effective not only for correcting specific symptoms but for placing the body in a state of overall balance. After a while, they provide a way of maintaining health that does not depend upon doctors or formalized medical care, but can be incorporated into any daily routine.

In addition to their physical benefits, certain yoga postures also operate on another level, in association with particular emotional states. For example, a series of postures referred to as "warrior poses" are especially vigorous and dynamic poses, requiring a good deal of strength to maintain. Their name is quite appropriate to their character, and a person experiencing the emotional quality of a warrior might physically express that feeling through these poses.

The relationship between emotional state and physical posture also goes the opposite way as well. Thus, holding a particular posture will tend to produce in a person the emotional state associated with that posture. As a result, if certain poses are practiced repeatedly, they may eventually create a subtle change in your usual emotional condition. Not only does the way you feel determine how you act, but the way you act also determines how you feel.

A person who holds himself with a curved spine, narrow slumped shoulders, head hung forward, and shallow respiration will typically be someone who has feelings of depression, self-consciousness, or low self-esteem. With an improved emotional state, that person will usually begin to stand up straighter, draw back the shoulders, and breathe more deeply. However, the intentional adoption of a better physical stance can, in itself, create a corresponding change in the emotional state. It is difficult to remain in a negative state when your physical posture reflects strength and stability.

The breath is often an especially good focus for beginning these changes. Feelings of anxiety or depression are typically accompanied by shallow, inhibited respiration, and the simple act of concentrating upon deeper and fuller breathing may produce a surprising change for the better in how one feels.

On a more metaphysical level, I wonder if the postures of yoga or the Taoist exercises of China have over time become charged with a special energy of their own. When

I practice one of the classical yoga postures, I sense a connection between myself and the millions of other individuals who, over thousands of years, have practiced this same posture to attain physical health and spiritual development. As each posture is held with as much concentration as possible, it is as though the combined concentration of so many others before me has transferred a certain power to these poses.

This practice constitutes a periodic balancing and cleansing of the body that can correct any imbalance before it becomes significant. When practiced regularly, other forms of physical exercise can have a similar effect. This is a critical consideration, because every disease has a beginning—a point where one imperceptibly slips from health into illness. Cancer begins with a single malignant cell, and a heart attack starts with only a small deposit on the wall of a blood vessel. At this stage, they may be easy to resolve if the body is stimulated to return to a state of balance, and they are caught before they become more complex problems.

The philosopher Lao-tzu says:

> Solve the small problem before it becomes big.
> The most involved fact in the world
> Could have been faced when it was simple,
> The biggest problem in the world
> Could have been solved when it was small.[1]

Whether this is accomplished through diet, exercise, spiritual practice, or any other approach available to us, this is perhaps the essence of how one maintains good health through life.

NOTE

1. Lao-tzu, *The Way of Life*, translated by Witter Bynner, (New York: Capricorn Books, 1962).

12

Medicine for
the Future

The Monopolization of Medicine

Throughout history, certain individuals have always been considered healers. Whether they are known as physicians, or by some other name, these people are recognized as possessing special skills for dealing with illness. The particular nature of their skills has inevitably reflected the nature of the society of which they have been a part.

Illness was once believed to be a consequence of supernatural powers or forces existing in the nonhuman realm. Therefore the task of the healer was quite different from what we expect of a doctor today. This healer appeased the offended spirit responsible for the illness, or drove out the evil forces inhabiting the body. A certain overlap existed between the province of the healer and that of the priest or religious leader. Although the role of healer undoubtedly involved a great deal of superstition, it also had the advantage of recognizing that physical illness is often related to psychological or spiritual events.

This is no longer the case today. The modern healer is not called upon to intercede for his patient in spiritual realms, but only to provide care on the physical level. Nevertheless, until fairly recently, Western culture in-

cluded a variety of healers who recognized some connection between illness and what was taking place in the
patient's whole life. At the turn of the century in America,
several types of medical pracititioners existed. These included allopaths, homeopaths, osteopaths, naturopaths,
and others. All offered different approaches to medical
treatment, and patients could choose among them.

The range of possible treatment available was considerable. Patients could be treated not only with synthetic
drugs or surgery, as they are today, but also with a variety
of herbs, mineral salts, homeopathic drugs, physical manipulation, hydrotherapy, or exercise, to name a few of the
more prominent techniques. Undoubtedly, a good deal of
quackery was involved in some of these practices, but a
sense of diversity existed, and an acceptance that there
was more than one way to practice medicine.

However, at the beginning of this century, all of this
changed. A movement arose to guarantee the quality of
medical care and protect the public by standardizing the
practice of medicine. One particular school of medicine,
called allopathic medicine, was established as the only
legitimate form of practice in America, and all other
schools of medicine were either largely eliminated or else
absorbed into this one.

The name "allopathic" is derived from the roots "allo,"
meaning other, and "path," meaning disease. Allopathy is
defined as ". . . a method of treating disease by inducing an
action opposite to the disease it is sought to cure." Thus,
an allopathic physician would treat a patient with a fever
by giving him a drug that would produce the opposite
effect and lower his temperature. What we now think of
as modern medicine is actually allopathic medicine, and
all physicians today are trained in this tradition.

This regulation of medical practice has done a lot to
preserve certain standards of treatment. It has eliminated
many worthless medical practices and helped to protect
patients against incompetent therapists or dangerous

treatments. However, it has also limited the opportunity to explore new ideas, and has created a situation in which a single profession holds almost complete authority over questions of health and illness. The result is the monolithic quality of established medicine that we find in the country today.

Medicine and Technology

The dominance of allopathic medicine has led to some drastic changes in how the role of the physician is defined. The doctor today is often perceived both by himself and by his patients as a sort of "supermechanic." Just as you bring your car to the garage when it is not running, you bring your body to the doctor to be fixed when you are sick. And in a disturbingly similar fashion, the parts of either one that are not working may be mechanically repaired, or, if necessary, removed.

This approach to illness has become characteristic of modern Western society. Medicine has embraced the enormous power of technology to provide quick and dramatic results, and this is the direction in which the mainstream of health care is moving today. As a result, technology has changed the face of medicine, so that much of what we do today would have seemed incredible to a doctor only a hundred years ago.

Imagine the reaction of a physician from the past to a heart transplant. What an extraordinary accomplishment this is, and what a complex technology is necessary to make it possible. Some see this as a glimpse of what the future of medicine will be like—a vision in which banks of organs are stored for routine replacement and most forms of disease have been conquered.

However, although there may be an element of truth to this vision, there is reason to believe that in some respects we are approaching the limits of technological solutions. While extremely impressive as a scientific achievement, heart transplants may prove to be not a taste of the future, but one of the more dramatic expressions of an approach that is reaching a point of diminishing returns.

Heart transplants are an especially powerful illustration of both the possibilities of medical technology and its limitations. They may be a remarkable life-saving measure for the few people who receive them successfully, but they are not a realistic solution to our medical problems on a large scale. If for no other reason, the future application of heart transplants is limited by financial considerations. We cannot expect to give a new heart to everyone with heart problems because it is simply not affordable.

The same is true of other technological innovations. We assume that every person should have access to the full range of modern medical care, yet the cost of making this care available is becoming unmanageable. The budget for health care is already astronomical, and it increases every year.

This increase in medical costs tends to follow a characteristic pattern. A new form of technology is introduced and found useful. It is then decided that this new technology must be made available to all patients. Implementing this decision adds still another new charge to the already huge health care bill.

A good example of this can be found in recent developments in X-ray technology. Doctors no longer rely only on ordinary X-rays, but now have available remarkable new techniques for looking inside the body. One of the most popular of these is the computerized tomographic scan, abbreviated as the CT-scan. This is a wonderful device that provides information in much more detail than can be obtained from ordinary X-rays. However, it is also very expensive.

Once the CT-scanner was introduced, doctors and hospitals everywhere were impressed with what it could do and wanted access to one. Within a short time, even small-town hospitals were getting their own scanners. As more and more hospitals became equipped with the necessary machinery, and doctors began making regular use of them, another very substantial expense was tacked onto the cost of medical care. While doctors managed to practice medicine only a few years ago without CT-scans, they now find them necessary in many situations.

As a practicing physician there are times when I find CT-scans extremely useful, and I appreciate that such technology exists. However, once they are routinely available, it is easy to order them more often than is really necessary, or even to use them in inappropriate situations. And, of course, once a hospital has spent all that money to purchase a CT-scanner, it is anxious to see this machinery used to pay back its investment. The result is that the patient winds up with a five-hundred-dollar CT-scan on his medical bill, when a fifty-dollar X-ray, or perhaps nothing at all, might have done as well.

In a hundred other areas of medicine, the same thing is taking place. But it cannot go on forever. We have reached, or will soon reach, the point where further developments are limited by their high cost. We will be forced to recognize that resources for increasingly expensive solutions to medical problems are no longer available, and at least some people may have no choice but to do without them.

Many people feel a real resistance to this idea because at first glance it seems to demand a compromise of the quality of available care. Actually, it may lead to changes in health care that could prove quite positive. A medical system that must rely a little less on expensive technology will be obliged to take another look at simpler and more natural solutions to maintaining health. And for modern medicine, that would be a very welcome perspective.

Although technological developments have been responsible for remarkable accomplishments in medicine, they have been pursued to the neglect of other concerns. The result is a system that has gone too far in one direction and must be brought back into balance. Despite all the achievements of modern medicine, it has still not been successful in creating a genuinely healthy society.

Alternatives in Medicine

We are now experiencing an attempt to restore greater balance to our medical system. As the mainstream of medicine moves ever further toward high-technology answers, another movement in a different direction is taking place. Heart transplants make headlines in the newspapers, but this movement is occurring more quietly, beneath the surface. It consists of people who are seeking answers to their health problems outside of conventional medicine. They are doing this because they are not satisfied with the care offered by their doctor. And there seem to be an increasingly large number of such people. These are not oddballs or health faddists. They are ordinary people concerned about their health, who are prepared to look wherever they must to find the care they need.

In response to this desire for another approach to health care, a great variety of "alternative" therapists have appeared. These include acupuncturists, psychotherapists, counselors, massage therapists, nutritionists, herbalists, and a variety of other therapists who often operate outside the mainstream of conventional medicine. This has added a new element of choice to health care that is slightly reminiscent of the situation that existed before medicine became so thoroughly dominated by allopathic physicians.

The movement toward what is called "alternative" or "holistic" medicine is a diverse one. It encompasses many philosophies and people, including a fair number of physicians. Undoubtedly it includes a good share of quacks, as well as occasional people of real genius, and everything in between. What all of these alternative practitioners share is an interest in alternatives to conventional treatment. As established medicine moves further toward one extreme, this movement toward the opposite polarity is growing in response.

The reaction of the medical profession toward this new interest in alternatives has generally not been positive. Physicians are often resistant to anything not taught in medical school, and tend to assume it is at best irrelevant, or at worst quackery.

A good example of this attitude is the response of the medical profession to the introduction of acupuncture in this country. Acupuncture is a safe, effective form of treatment that should be a legitimate part of health care, but its origins are strange and unfamiliar. It is not a new treatment developed by a modern research laboratory, but a technique handed down from an ancient and foreign culture. Thus, rather than seriously examining acupuncture, the reaction has been to hold it at arm's length. While not entirely rejecting it, organized medicine has labeled it indefinitely as "experimental," and holds it in a sort of limbo.

Yet despite this unenthusiastic reception, acupuncture has taken hold in this country. People are interested in whatever can really help them, so that acupuncture has become fairly widely practiced, although usually not by doctors. A few physicians have pursued an individual interest in acupuncture, but its practice has by default been left largely to others.

Although many nonphysician acupuncturists are quite expert, it seems unfortunate for the practice of acupuncture to be so separated from the rest of medicine. Physicians have limited the scope of what they are able to provide their patients, and because they are unlikely to refer patients to someone who is not another physician, a valuable treatment is largely excluded from conventional medicine. The same is often true of other alternative approaches.

Combining Conventional and Alternative Medicine

Many patients are reluctant even to tell their doctor that they are seeing another therapist for some less conventional treatment, because they are afraid of his reaction. And this skepticism of physicians toward alternative therapists is frequently returned in kind. This is an unfortunate situation, because both groups could learn much from each other and actually complement each other's work.

Many nonphysician therapists seem to have the time and willingness to form personal relationships with patients, which can be a very important part of any treatment. They are often prepared to deal with people as individuals, and to relate their medical symptoms to what is going on in their lives. However, they do not have the physician's knowledge and training in the functioning of the body and the diagnosis of disease. With the best of intentions, they may sometimes get involved in problems that really require the expertise of a physician.

On the other hand, doctors do have the knowledge and technical skills, but they are often unwilling to explore simple, natural approaches to health or examine the individual lives of their patients. In many cases, a combination of what both have to offer may prove most effective.

In my practice, I have tried to serve as a bridge between the established framework of conventional medicine and the alternative therapists who work outside of this framework. One physician cannot provide everything for every patient, so it is helpful to work with other people who have different skills to offer. Doctors routinely refer patients to other medical specialists, and there is no reason why help cannot be found outside the medical profession as well.

I have learned a good deal from working with various therapists whose work will not be found in any medical school curriculum. They, in turn, have appreciated the opportunity to use their skills in the context of a professional medical practice, with the supervision of a physician available.

For several years, my office staff included a massage therapist, a yoga therapist who worked with exercise and breath, and a nurse who trained patients in guided imagery and relaxation. After evaluating a new patient, I could ask one or more of them to become involved, depending upon what treatment seemed most appropriate.

Occasionally, all four of us would work with the same patient. This could be extremely effective, and provided the opportunity to approach the existing problem from several perspectives at once. With a number of therapists involved, the patient was far more likely to make a personal connection with at least one of us, and this connection would be especially helpful to the patient's recovery.

Unfortunately, such forms of therapy are often viewed by physicians as not being "real medicine," but merely frills that can never produce the results that drugs or surgery can achieve. Yet they are not frills at all. They can be powerful, effective techniques. I have repeatedly seen people who had been unresponsive to years of conventional treatment respond well to these alternatives. Helping to modify how a person eats, how he breathes, how he moves and holds his body, or how he reacts emotionally to different situations is a fundamental aspect of real healing. Working on this level, one can address the aspects of daily living that underlie whatever illness exists.

This work can also do more than just resolve a particular medical problem. By giving people a better understanding of their physical or emotional patterns, it can lead to changes that extend throughout their lives. These changes can continue long after the specific complaint that brought the patient to the office is gone, and be helpful in preventing similar problems in the future. This is what doctors are really supposed to be doing—leading people to changes in their lives that will create a lasting improvement in health.

I welcome other therapists in my practice, and I am delighted to be able to offer their services to patients. What is perhaps most satisfying is to provide these services to people who would normally not have contact with such alternatives. Some patients would never think of having a massage or attending a yoga class or practicing self-relaxation. These are simply not activities that are part of their cultural background. And even if they thought of doing them, they would not know where to begin.

But in the context of the doctor's office, all of these practices become quite acceptable. If I tell someone as his doctor that I would like him to see the massage therapist or the yoga therapist in the office, there is no problem at all. And once he has gone for the first time, he will see for himself how useful it can be and need no further convincing.

It should be up to doctors to assume the lead in making the services of other health care providers available— certainly there is nobody better qualified to do it. But doctors have interpreted their role as leaders as one of excluding whatever is unfamiliar. It would be refreshing to see the medical profession abandon this narrow viewpoint and open to the exciting possibilities that exist for helping patients to get well.

Rather than condemning what they do not fully understand, or what seems a bit strange, physicians could take responsibility for blending different therapies into the mainstream of medicine. In this way, they could best assure that when such therapies were used, they were done so in an intelligent and professional fashion. This is the direction in which medical care must move in the future in order to provide people with help that really addresses their needs.

Balancing the Polarities

Although the medical profession receives a lot of criticism today, most individual physicians really want to help their patients. When they provide care that does not deal with the real causes of illness, it is not only unsatisfying for the patient but for the doctor as well. Yet I am continually dismayed by how I see medicine being practiced. Many doctors provide care that is so lacking in an intuitive sense of what is happening with their patients that it simply cannot be the best of which they are capable.

Often doctors seem trapped in a routine that is difficult to change. They may realize that what they are doing for their patients is not really the answer, but they have become so engrossed in the daily demands of their work they have no time for alternatives.

In a sense, our medical system is suffering from an illness; its symptoms are the problems that modern medicine faces. Financial costs of health care are growing unmanageable, with no control in sight; doctors are overwhelmed with legal regulations and the mountains of paperwork they entail; patients are suing their doctors more than ever before, so that doctors must practice with one eye over their shoulder for malpractice claims. And most of all, despite its success in some areas, our medical system is simply not providing effective help with the medical problems people are experiencing today.

Just as in an individual with an illness, these symptoms are an indication that changes must be made to restore a normal balance to the system. Medicine is an art as well as a science. But while the scientific element of medicine is much in evidence, the other half of this dual nature is often ignored. Thus, that side of human experience that cannot be strictly weighed and measured, and that can only be appreciated by the artist, is frequently excluded from consideration.

When a person gets well, for example, because it has been suggested that this will happen, the outcome cannot be explained in terms of "scientific" medicine. Therefore, it is given a convenient label and then largely ignored. The physician as scientist does not know quite what to make of this phenomenon, but the physician as artist can make good use of it in the practice of medicine.

The terms "left brain" and "right brain" have recently become a popular shorthand for expressing these two perspectives. The two halves of the brain each have characteristic mental processes; in very simple terms, the left brain is the scientific half—logical, rational, and linear in its concepts—while the right brain is the more artistic half, more concerned with the total image or concept. Each of the two is appropriate for certain situations, but when one dominates consistently to the exclusion of the other, the result may be a limited, unbalanced way of thinking.

It is primarily left brain thinking that is encouraged in physicians. Thus the sometimes nonrational aspects of human life must either be explained in terms comprehensible to the left brain or simply ignored.

In the movement toward alternatives in health care, a more "right-brain" form of thinking is often encountered. This may involve a willingness to work on a more intuitive level and make use of treatment that cannot be entirely explained in objective, scientific terms.

Alternative approaches provide a refreshing contrast to conventional medicine's preoccupation with hard, cold measurement. However, it is easy to go too far in this direction as well. Abandoning a scientific foundation entirely can leave one thoroughly adrift, with no sense of objective justification for anything that is done. A fusion of left and right brain perspectives is needed—a solid foundation of scientific analysis, combined with a willingness to accept the existence of more intuitive, nonrational aspects of life.

The Qualities of a Physician

Although modern medicine has largely been the province of men, certain aspects of the healing experience have traditionally belonged to women. One sign of medicine moving toward a greater balance has been the inclusion of more women as physicians. However, there is still no clear sense of what these women are now expected to contribute to medicine.

To be successfully accepted as physicians, women are expected to be just as logical, rational, and scientific as their male colleagues, if not more so. Although this does create a more equitable balance of the sexes, it does not make for any real change in medicine. What we need is not more *women* in medicine, but more of the *feminine* principle. Women physicians who think and act in precisely the same way as men do will not make a difference.

By the feminine principle, I mean the intuitive capacity that is attuned to the perceptions and processes of the right brain. While these characteristics are more commonly associated with women, they exist in men as well, although their expression by either men or women is usually discouraged in the medical profession. When the feminine side does appear in medicine, it generally takes a secondary role.

We accept that doctors are usually male, while nurses are female. It is the nurse who is allowed the nurturing, feminine characteristics not permitted to the doctor. It is considered quite normal for your hospital nurse to give you a back rub the night before surgery. But can anyone imagine the surgeon coming in instead to give you the back rub himself? The very idea seems incongruous in terms of the behavior we expect from doctors.

This lack of balance in what is expected of doctors is reflected in the lack of balance that exists throughout our medical system. A critical place to begin changing this system is at the level of how the individual physician approaches the practice of medicine. The physician as healer is composed of various parts. He or she is not only a scientist, but also includes aspects of the artist, of the priest or priestess, and perhaps even the magician.

To function as a physician is to pursue a role of many possible dimensions, but the practice of medicine today has unfortunately been defined in such a way that its potential is unnecessarily limited. Powerful resources for healing exist within each individual and in the world around us. Too often they are neglected by modern medicine, although they may be utilized by the physician who is willing to open his own perceptions, and acknowledge the existence of these alternatives.

A New Direction in Medicine

All the problems that exist in medicine today have the potential to be solved creatively—to restore a sense of innovation to the practice of medicine and make it more satisfying for both doctors and patients. For this to happen, we must be willing to change some of the ways in which we approach the issues of personal health and illness. Perhaps most importantly, we need to recognize that many serious medical problems are not amenable to successful treatment by external intervention with drugs or surgery. They cannot be solved by developing still more elaborate and expensive technology, but only by individuals taking responsibility for their own health. This involves the prevention of disease through attention to such things as appropriate diet and personal habits, regular physical exercise, and effective management of emotional stress.

We must also recognize that when illness does occur, it does so for a reason. Thus, although it may be necessary to treat the symptoms of an illness, it is also essential to discover and address the reason for these symptoms. Only in this way can we appreciate the real cause of illness, and understand what can be done, either physically or emotionally, to try to resolve it. It is up to the doctor not only to treat the symptoms, but to help the patient realize why they exist and how best to respond to them.

This approach to health care places a great deal of responsibility on the individual both for prevention and treatment of illness, but this is as it should be. Ultimately we are each responsible for our own well-being. We cannot expect doctors to assume this responsibility for us. What doctors *can* do is offer additional help, when needed, in our own efforts to recover and maintain good health.

Modern drugs and technology provide essential help at times of serious illness, and are a fundamental part of our health-care system. However, their use is over-emphasized today. In many situations they are neither appropriate nor effective, and something else is needed. Other techniques of treatment exist that do not involve external agents, but act by stimulating the body's own mechanisms of healing and self-regulation to function more effectively. These include psychological techniques involving elements of hypnosis or suggestion, physical treatments such as acupuncture, counseling in diet and nutrition, and still others. These all share the property that they do not so much treat disease as they encourage health. Their use reflects a somewhat different way of thinking about health and illness, and points to a new direction in which medicine can move.

By taking greater individual responsibility, it is possible for any of us to achieve a more positive level of personal health. And by providing care that addresses the real causes of illness, it is possible for doctors to give their patients the help they need to maintain this health.

Annotated Bibliography

An enormous number of books are available to read further on the various subjects considered here. I have selected a few for specific mention that may be particularly interesting or helpful.

Arms, Suzanne. *Immaculate Deception*. Boston: Houghton Mifflin, 1975. Examines the problems associated with modern, technological childbirth and how they might be avoided.

Bailey, Covert. *Fit or Fat*. Boston: Houghton Mifflin, 1978. A popular book about exercising properly to maintain physical fitness and optimal body weight.

Ballentine, Rudolph, M.D. *Diet and Nutrition: A Holistic Approach*. Honesdale, PA: The Himalayan International Institute, 1978. A large, well-written book combining Eastern and Western concepts of nutrition. If you were to read just one book on diet, this would be an excellent choice.

Bliss, Shepherd, ed. *The New Holistic Health Handbook*. Lexington, MA: Stephen Greene Press, 1985. An extensive survey and resource guide for holistic health care.

Bresler, David E. *Free Yourself from Pain*. New York: Simon & Schuster, 1979. Examines a wide variety of alternative approaches to the treatment of chronic pain.

Drury, Neville, ed. *Inner Health: The Health Benefits of Relaxation, Meditation and Visualization*. San Leandro, CA: Prism Press, 1985. A collection by various therapists working in this field.

Fields, Rick, et al. *Chop Wood, Carry Water: A Guide to Finding Spiritual Fulfillment in Everyday Life*. Los Angeles: J. P. Tarcher, 1984. A resource book that touches on many areas related to health.

Gawain, Shakti. *Creative Visualization*. Mill Valley, CA: Whatever Publishing, 1978. A guide to utilizing the power of positive visualization in your life.

Hewitt, James. *The Complete Yoga Book*. New York: Schocken Books, 1977. Many other good books are also available on the subject of yoga. This one provides a very comprehensive overview of the theory and practice of yoga.

Joy, W. Brugh, M.D. *Joy's Way*. Los Angeles: J. P. Tarcher, 1979. An exploration by a physician of the possibilities of healing with body energies.

Kaptchuk, Ted. *The Web That Has No Weaver*. New York: Congdon and Weed, 1983. Examines the philosophy and practice of traditional acupuncture and Oriental medicine.

Levine, Stephen. *Who Dies?* Garden City, NY: Anchor Press/ Doubleday, 1982. Stephen Levine has written several powerful books on how we can approach the issues of death and dying.

Pelletier, Kenneth R. *Holistic Medicine*. New York: Dell, 1977. Dr. Pelletier is also the author of several other well-documented books on stress-related illness, mind/body interactions, and the general subject of holistic medicine.

Pritikin, Nathan. *The Pritikin Program for Diet and Exercise*. New York: Bantam Books, 1979. This book and several others by Nathan Pritikin have been influential in popularizing the benefits of a low-fat diet based on complex carbohydrates.

Swami Rama; Ballentine, Rudolph, M.D.; and Swami Ajaya. *Yoga and Psychotherapy*. Honesdale, PA.: Himalayan International Institute, 1976. A fascinating examination of Eastern concepts of health and psychotherapy in terms accessible to a Western reader.

Reich, Wilhelm. *Selected Writings: An Introduction to Orgonomy*. New York: Farrar, Straus & Giroux, 1951. Selections from the extensive work of Wilhelm Reich.

Robertson, Laurel, et al. *Laurel's Kitchen*. New York: Bantam Books, 1976. The encyclopedia of natural foods and vegetarian cooking. Includes a great deal of basic nutritional information as well as a large selection of recipes.

Simonton, O. Carl, M.D. *Getting Well Again*. New York: Bantam Books, 1980. A pioneering book on the use of visual imagery in the treatment of cancer.

Weil, Andrew, M.D. *Health and Healing*. Boston: Houghton Mifflin, 1983. Examines alternative approaches to health care. Dr. Weil is also the author of several other interesting books in related areas.

Books and Tapes

Additional copies of *In Search of Health*, as well as the following casette tapes by Dr. Volen, are available from Gateway Press.

DEEP RELAXATION   Michael Volen, M.D.

This tape leads the listener through a gradual, progressive relaxation exercise for the entire body. It is designed to help relieve physical tension or emotional stress, and can also be used at bedtime to help with difficulty in sleeping.

UNDERSTANDING YOUR SYMPTOMS Michael Volen, M.D.

In order to resolve the symptoms of illness, it is often necessary to understand what their presence is telling you. This tape begins by establishing a receptive state of relaxation, then leads you through a guided communication with your own symptoms.

These tapes are a good way to put into practice some of the ideas presented in this book. However, they should not be considered a substitute for consultation with a physician for any medical problems.

In Search of Health (Book)	$8.95
Deep Relaxation (Cassette Tape)	$12.50
Understanding Your Symptoms (Cassette Tape)	$12.50

Postage and Handling: $1.75 for the first book or tape, plus $0.35 for each additional item.

To order, list the books or tapes you wish to receive, with your name and address. Please send your check, including postage and handling, plus 6% sales tax (if California resident), to:

Gateway Press
P.O. Box 5180
Mill Valley, CA 94942

Inquiries for bulk orders are also invited.